CRITICAL HEALTH AND LEARNING DISABILITIES

This empirically grounded book presents a critical, interdisciplinary perspective on social and cultural issues related to the health and wellbeing of people with learning disabilities. Through an exploration of healthcare, love and intimacy, pregnancy and childbirth, housing, employment and food the book highlights the enduringly impoverished lives and premature deaths people labelled with learning disabilities experience globally and suggests that such structural violence amounts to social murder.

Through the lens of critical disability studies, the book links the debates around learning disabilities to the larger framework of deinstitutionalisation. It takes a closer look at the label "learning disability", which remains associated with stigma and shame, and advances comprehension of how and why it is that the lives of this group of people are systematically constrained and shortened. The book further identifies recommendations that can be utilised for challenging and changing these circumstances.

It is essential reading for those involved in social and cultural issues related to the lives of people with learning disabilities, and also beneficial for advanced students in sociology, anthropology, psychology, allied health sciences and other related disciplines. It will also be valuable for researchers and health and social care professionals seeking critical insights about their work.

Sara Ryan is a Professor of Social Care at the Manchester Metropolitan University. Her main research interests are experiences of exclusion and marginalisation, particularly in relation to learning disabilities and autism, and strategies of resistance, activism and advocacy.

Critical Approaches to Health

The Routledge *Critical Approaches to Health* series aims to present critical, interdisciplinary books around psychological, social and cultural issues related to health. Each volume in the series provides a critical approach to a particular issue or important topic, and is of interest and relevance to students and practitioners across the social sciences. The series is produced in association with the International Society of Critical Health Psychology (ISCHP).

Series Editors: Kerry Chamberlain & Antonia Lyons

Titles in the series:

Medical Humanities
Ethics, Aesthetics, Politics
Alan Bleakley

Making Mental Health
A Global History
Elizabeth Roberts-Pedersen

Critical approaches to death, dying and bereavement
Erica Borgstrom and Renske Visser

Critical Health and Learning Disabilities
An Exploration of Erasure and Social Murder
Sara Ryan

For more information about this series, please visit: www.routledge.com/Critical-Approaches-to-Health/book-series/CRITHEA

"When I say that the first chapter is called, '*As natural as the air around us'; the social murder of people labelled with learning disabilities*, you begin to understand the necessary violence of this book. The book punctures all our various excuses and complicit and ineffective endeavours that have failed to bring about change. It's urgent and passionate and above all utterly human – a quality which should go without saying but, as the book so forensically exposes, seems to need saying again.

Everything gets 'turned over' in this book, things get called out – theory, eugenics, ableism, health and care systems, governments, academia, charities. There is an unassailable and deeply uncomfortable and provocative argument at the core of this book about a State-sanctioned and State-actioned refusal to see learning disabled people as 'proper people' at all.

People being denied citizenship, denied life, denied love. Systematically, casually, deliberately. It made me want to cry tears of anger and deep, deep sadness, see my own part in it all and then get on with trying to be a useful ally. That the book is so badly needed is a terrible indictment. The question it leaves me with is, what now? It cannot be more of the same."

Professor David Abbott, *Chair in Social Policy, University of Bristol*

"This compelling book lays bare the stark reality of how the humanity of people with learning disabilities is so often denied. By centering the concept of 'social murder,' the book reveals the conditions that lead to diminished lives and deaths, which remain disturbingly ignored by both wider society and those in power. Sara carefully guides readers through this frightening and incomprehensible landscape, posing critical questions about why so many scholars, policy makers and systems continue to overlook the lives of people with learning disabilities. This is an important read for all those committed to exposing the structural violence at play in the lives of people with learning disabilities."

Professor Katherine Runswick-Cole,
Chair in Education, University of Sheffield

"In this hard-hitting book, Professor Ryan uses exceptionally wide research to lay bare the scandalous way we treat people with learning disabilities – as people less deserving of respect, health, wealth or even life. It is a must read for people who care about human rights, as a prelude to changing this scandal."

Jan Walmsley, *Visiting Professor of the History of Learning Disabilities, The Open University*

CRITICAL HEALTH AND LEARNING DISABILITIES

An Exploration of Erasure and Social Murder

Sara Ryan

Routledge
Taylor & Francis Group
LONDON AND NEW YORK

Designed cover image: getty images via SEAN GLADWELL

First published 2026
by Routledge
4 Park Square, Milton Park, Abingdon, Oxon OX14 4RN

and by Routledge
605 Third Avenue, New York, NY 10158

Routledge is an imprint of the Taylor & Francis Group, an informa business

British Library Cataloguing-in-Publication Data
A catalogue record for this book is available from the British Library

ISBN: 9781032644844 (hbk)
ISBN: 9781032605005 (pbk)
ISBN: 9781032644868 (ebk)

DOI: 10.4324/9781032644868

Typeset in Times New Roman
by Newgen Publishing UK

CONTENTS

SERIES EDITOR PREFACE

Critical Approaches to Health

Health is a major issue for people all around the world, and is fundamental to individual wellbeing, personal achievements and satisfaction, as well as to families, communities and societies. It is also embedded in social notions of participation and citizenship. Much has been written about health, from a variety of perspectives and disciplines, but a lot of this writing takes a biomedical and positivist approach to health matters, neglecting the historical, social and cultural contexts and environments within which health is experienced, understood and practiced. We developed this series of books to offer critical social science perspectives on important, relevant and timely health topics.

The Critical Approaches to Health series provides new writing on health by presenting books that offer critical, interdisciplinary and theoretical writing about health, where matters of health are framed quite broadly. The series seeks to include books ranging across important health matters, including general health-related issues (such as gender and media), major social issues for health (such as medicalisation, obesity and palliative care), particular health concerns (such as pain, doctor-patient interaction, health services and health technologies), particular health problems (such as diabetes, autoimmune disease and medically unexplained illness), or health for specific groups of people (such as the health of migrants, the homeless and the aged), or combinations of these.

The series seeks above all to promote critical thought about health matters. By critical, we mean going beyond the critique of the topic and work in the field, to more general considerations of power and benefit, and in particular, to addressing concerns about whose understandings and interests are upheld and whose are marginalised by the approaches, findings and practices in these various domains of health. Such critical agendas involve reflections on what constitutes knowledge, how it is created and how it is used. Accordingly, critical approaches consider epistemological and theoretical positioning, as well as issues of methodology and practice, and seek to examine how health is enmeshed within broader social relations and structures. Books within this series take up this challenge and seek to provide new insights and understandings by applying a critical agenda to their topics. Explore the previous books in the series at www.routledge.com/Critical-Approaches-to-Health/book-series/CRITHEA

This book, *Critical Health and Learning Disabilities: An Exploration of Erasure and Social Murder*, is hard-hitting. Sara Ryan takes the reader on a tour de force, delivering a compelling – and at times extremely uncomfortable and challenging – account of the ways in which people with learning disabilities are marginalised and excluded, their experiences discounted and ignored and how this leads to their social murder – their premature and preventable deaths. The argument is incredibly powerful and unwavering throughout, right from Chapter 1, where Ryan asserts that an exploration "of the theoretical and philosophical debates and positions in relation to learning disabilities [reveals that this] area remains shrouded in ignorance, assumptions, confusion and prejudice which, when layers are stripped away, reveals a mix of duplicity, deceit and collusion".

Throughout the book, Ryan demonstrates how epistemic ignorance leads to profound forms of epistemic injustice. She convincingly demonstrates how swathes of people from different spheres (including researchers, policymakers, carers, charities, governments and others) have shown, and continue to show, ignorance of the learning disabled world and people with learning disabilities, whether intentionally or unintentionally. This includes knowledge that they have but do not act on, knowledge that they do not have but should have, and knowledge that they refuse to have. Misunderstanding, ignoring and refusing to know about the lives and experiences of people with learning disabilities, despite countless governmental reviews, inquiries, academic articles, books, policies, information and so on, leads Ryan to conclude that social murder "is happening in full view".

This book is a call to arms. The ongoing, systemic and appalling failure to treat people with learning disabilities as people who live, love and enjoy, is conveyed across key areas of life. This includes their personal relationships, loving relationships, sexual relationships, health and healthcare, housing and employment, food and eating and their citizenship. And while research is conducted about people with learning disabilities in each of these areas, they are mostly not included as participants themselves, with assumptions made that they cannot participate, they do not have anything of value to contribute, that it is too challenging to include them, that ethics review boards will not let them participate. Ryan asks why researchers are not redesigning their research and figuring out ways of engagement, so that people with learning disabilities can be included and contribute to the knowledge that is gathered about them? The status quo, as Ryan convincingly demonstrates, is a form of structural discrimination and violence.

This book is at times a distressing read, being ultimately about human rights, who they are and are not afforded to, and who is colluding in human rights abuses. We all – researchers, medical professionals, policymakers, charities and anyone engaged in this field – need to be thinking much more critically about people with learning disabilities and our responsibilities for and towards them, and consider how complicit we are in both disavowing the ordinary aspects of everyday life and othering people with learning disabilities. Ryan sincerely and compassionately discusses the urgent need for moral courage, rather than moral bystanding, to end the brutal dismissing and discounting of the experiences, feelings, perceptions and knowledge of people with learning disabilities.

Antonia Lyons and Kerry Chamberlain
February 2025

ACKNOWLEDGEMENTS

This book became something more than a book at some point over the last 12 months. It began as a dogged and loosely organised academic attempt to record and make sense of what has been researched and written about people labelled with learning disabilities under a framework of health inequalities, drawing on published research, reports and enquiries. It soon extended to personal and professional experiences, friendships, life and relationships. Given what this focus generated, it became a complicated, sometimes insomnia inducing labour of love, anger and intense sadness that involved essential contributions from others. I want to thank Janet Read for her consistent and unwavering support and kindness from my pup days as a doctoral student twenty odd years ago, to staunch #JusticeForLB campaigner and textile artist, and meeting at a mid-point between our homes in Stafford last autumn to lose ourselves in a warm cafe for hours to deal with the work of putting me on a track of owning this [shared] writing endeavour and doing it better. George Julian, journalist, co-plotter and key #JusticeForLB campaigner spent chunks of the Christmas break providing feedback and knowledge based on her unparalleled work documenting and curating the atrocities people and their families have experienced over the last decade or so. I have no idea how George does this painstaking and comprehensive work which is slowly having a visible impact on the workings of coronial processes in the UK and wider. I want to thank my newish home in the Department of Social Care and Social Work at Manchester Metropolitan University, Jenny Fisher, Chris Hatton and the members of our small and imperfectly formed *Learning Disabilities and Autism Research Group* for the support, warmth, activist and academic commitment, discussion, collaboration and enthusiasm for monthly chips and curry sauce. To the *Flourishing Lives* tour team of Beth Richards, Rebecca Spalding, Alan Spalding and the indomitable Angeli Vaid, and friends and colleagues at My Life My Choice, I want to say thank you for your commitment, honesty, enthusiasm and kindness. To editors Antonia Lyons and Kerry Chamberlain, thank you for making this process peaceful and supportive. Finally, to my partner Richard Huggins who has walked alongside this book before it was even a thing, across countless beautiful Peak District walks with our dog Sid, always ready to discuss issues, think about, develop and offer careful thoughts, insights, ideas and arguments with generosity, unwavering support, righteous anger and love, thank you.

1

'AS NATURAL AS THE AIR AROUND US'

The social murder of people labelled with learning disabilities

Introduction: the landscape

People labelled with learning disabilities experience impoverished lives globally and continue to die prematurely. Layers of social injustice are baked into obscurity as people are subjected to structural violence, that is, harm as an often-invisible manifestation of inequalities of power, resources and opportunities (Medvedyuk et al 2021). Structural violence has been described as:

> ... silent, it does not show – it is essentially static, it is the tranquil waters. In a static society, personal violence will be registered, whereas structural violence may be seen as about as natural as the air around us.
>
> *(Galtung 1973 p111)*

This book aims to demonstrate how structural and other forms of violence directed at people with learning disabilities do show. They are documented, curated, published and discussed in government-funded inquiries, independent reviews and safeguarding inquiries. They are explicit in research publications, though not necessarily recognised as such by researchers, and outlined in regulatory reports and sometimes wider media coverage. Because the humanity of people with learning disabilities is too often denied or contested, this violence is not recognised as violence and is read as acceptable. If you are not considered human, legislative protections underpinned by statutory criminal justice systems and processes, and the legal and other mechanisms generated by obligations to human rights frameworks and treaties, do not apply in ways we might expect. I demonstrate how

DOI: 10.4324/9781032644868-1

a range of stakeholders, including politicians, coroners, judges, commissioners, health and social care professionals, providers, support workers and sometimes family carers engage in manipulation to sustain this violence which cannot be explained as benign.

While recent work theorises the link between austerity measures and structural violence (see, for example, Kiely and Warnock 2023), I argue the premature and often preventable deaths of people with learning disabilities in Global North countries represent a collective and longstanding form of social murder because the foreseeable and avoidable conditions that precipitate these deaths remain untroubled, reported and repeatedly ignored (Engels 1845, Grover 2019).

Let us take as one example the Learning from Lives and Deaths Review (LEDER) programme established in England in 2017 after a series of reports and inquiries revealed people with learning disabilities were dying nearly 30 years before their non-disabled peers. Funded by the Department of Health and Social Care, the programme reports annually on the premature deaths of people with learning disabilities. While I return to the implementation of this programme in Chapter 2, here I highlight the latest LEDER report found 42% of deaths reviewed were deemed avoidable (White et al 2023). A decade earlier, the Confidential Inquiry into the Premature Deaths of People with Learning Disabilities which led to the establishment of the LEDER programme found 48% of deaths were avoidable and 42% premature (Heslop et al 2013). The lack of effective action in the face of this well-rehearsed knowledge, of knowing people will *die* as an outcome of certain and repeated conditions, constitutes social murder.

The living and working conditions Engels (1845) identified as the cause of the premature deaths of working-class people nearly 200 years ago are largely incorporated into what are now called the social determinants of health (Commission on Social Determinants of Health 2008, Medvedyuk et al 2021). Systemic, unjust and enduring inequalities, which include higher rates of poverty, decreased access to: affordable and appropriate housing; accessible, safe transportation; and appropriate and timely healthcare (Emerson and Hatton 2014). The impact of these inequalities is deeply inscribed on people's minds and bodies.

People with learning disabilities face further and again enduring biases among, for example, healthcare professionals which include discriminatory attitudes, negative assumptions about people's capacity to be involved in their healthcare, instances of pain not being believed, disrespectfulness and resistance to making reasonable adjustments (Gréaux et al 2023). People with learning disabilities are more likely to be victims of abuse, violence and hate crime or 'disablist violence' (Daly and Smith 2022) while few cases reach the bar of criminal prosecution. These negative experiences are amplified by intersectional characteristics and identities which include disability, gender, ethnicity, sexuality, place and socio-economic status (Goodley 2023, Hassiotis 2020, Miner et al 2024, Yee et al 2018). People with learning disabilities continue to experience structural exclusion and discrimination as they are systematically obstructed from being part of and contributing to everyday life.

> This is a minority that is excluded even from the idea that outgroups can challenge their own marginalisation – they are excluded from the ingroup of outgroups, so to speak.
>
> *(Goodey 2017 p27)*

I explore throughout this book how Goodey's extreme positioning is justifiably articulated; how broad markers of social determinants of health sit peculiarly with contradictions, complexities and sometimes absurdities in relation to the lives of people with learning disabilities. That is, people who are consistently subjected to treatment and experiences that explicitly contravene legislation which in England includes the Human Rights Act (1998), Mental Capacity Act (2005) and Equality Act (2010); in Sweden, the Ormsorgslag of 1986 and Law of Support and Service (1994); and in the United States, the Americans with Disabilities Act (1995). A timeline of policy failures in England offers graphic illustration of repeatedly broken promises (see https://reignitingdebate.blogs.bristol.ac.uk/). Legislative requirements are not met and day-to-day access to support is delayed, deferred and diverted through 'banal' techniques of neglect, interpreted as institutional neglect, a form of structural violence;

> Each act of institutional neglect – each avoided phone call or unfair discharge – might seem insignificant. But writ large across the declining institutions of the British welfare state, these instances combine to power a grinding down and wearing out of marginalised bodies which, with its gradual tempo, barely registers in a popular consciousness oriented towards the spectacular.
>
> *(Kiely and Warnock 2023 p332)*

Severe material deprivation resulting from the lack of access to opportunities, to being understood, respected and seen as human, is further accepted and ignored in countries which have signed up to or ratified human rights frameworks. The fundamental aspirational strands of these frameworks are unfulfilled and ignored. People with learning disabilities experience appalling treatment, which extends from the seemingly light touch like avoided phone calls to long-term torture and abuse. These contradictions have led to a critical focus in this book on what should be considered mundane and everyday aspects of everyday life, including family, community, love, sex and eating to explore what these experiences reveal about the material, social, political, economic and interpersonal factors that impact upon and shape people's lives.

I do not define the term 'learning disabilities' because I see it as socially constructed, that is, it is something that is made up. It is a label applied to children who fail developmental markers created by psy-disciplines such as psychology and psychiatry (Rose 1985). Once applied, these labels change the experience, shape and direction of children's lives and those of their families. Altermark (2017) presents a meticulous unpacking of the pathologisation of this label that does not need repeating here. Instead, I highlight one of his arguments that underpins much of what is discussed in this book; that the technologies used to describe the apparently independently existing condition [learning disabilities] work to manufacture that very condition. The "symptoms" of learning disability do not mean anything other than being a symptom of a thing called learning disabilities. In effect, the symptoms are the condition (Altermark 2017 p32).

Cluley et al (2020) suggest that while the existence of different terms for learning disabilities (developmental delay, intellectual disability and so on) is fine, a consistent philosophical starting point in representing the realities of being a person with learning disabilities is more useful in terms of generating relevant policy and practice than thinking about what a learning disability *is*. Drawing on and extending Hughes and Paterson's (1997) phenomenological articulation of disability, materiality and impairment, these authors suggest learning disability is:

> integral to how people with learning disabilities experience the world, in that it is lived as a bodily experience that is both felt and socially constructive, by virtue of the body's outward-facing orientation within the world.
>
> *(Cluley et al 2020 p242)*

For Cluley et al, this approach overrides the homogenisation, the grouping together, of people with learning disabilities apparent in social policy in various countries, including England, Canada and Australia. It allows consideration of bodies, materiality, intersectionality and specific histories of social interaction. I explore in Chapter 2 how this homogenisation and thereby discounting of experiences is further perpetuated by the wider academic community which often fails to critically reflect upon and interrogate, or even notice, the contributions it makes to the sustained oppression of people with learning disabilities.

My aim is to carefully pick through this often-incomprehensible landscape of what I describe and present as abhorrence, drawing on extensive research, policy and legislative developments to try to make some theoretical sense of what underpins this largely universal discounting of people with learning disabilities and what this discounting means. In the following chapters, I critically draw on research that often relies on orthodox understandings of learning disabilities, as people are defined by research and seen and treated in particular ways. I lean towards more recent scholarship where possible to develop a contemporary understanding of the so far marginalised field of learning disabilities studies. The views of people with learning disabilities from published research are included throughout, while acknowledging the troublesome evidence base of this literature which can rely on assumption rather than evidence-based practice and distorted scholarship (Medina 2018).

In this introductory chapter, I unpack what this orthodoxy means through exploring theoretical, philosophical debates and positions in relation to learning disabilities. This area remains shrouded in ignorance, assumptions, confusion and prejudice which, when layers are stripped away reveals a mix of duplicity, deceit and collusion. Even those individuals or groups you might expect to think critically about and engage with people with learning disabilities can fail to do so. It is important this landscape is presented clearly to allow the remainder of this book to be read, understood and appreciated in hopefully innovative ways.

Where to start?

Disability, as a material, political, social, discursive way of being, as a form of common and universal human variation (Garland-Thomson 2011), is a late arrival among activist and academic led social movements demanding equal rights and social justice. Indeed, there has been resistance to considering it at all. A brief look back at the early days of the American Sociological Association (ASA) and British Sociological Association (BSA), the formal membership groups of a discipline that claims to embody practices of enlightened thinking, forensic scrutiny of societal structures, systems and processes and the shape and colour of everyday life, shows how mainstream eugenic thinking and derogatory attitudes towards disability were. Disability has been unseen in spaces where it should be of key interest and learning disability remains in the dimmest distance.

A content analysis of a decade of the Proceedings of the American Sociological Society annual meetings (1906–1915) found disability was largely ignored and, when mentioned, vilified by academic presenters (Gerschick and Stevens 2016). This vilification was met by silence in the written commentary about the proceedings. In an early example of moral bystanding, an extraordinary list of analyses of American sociology is compiled in which disability is not mentioned *even* when the reviewers are explicitly seeking gaps in existing research.

> Thus, within the discipline of sociology the intellectual history of disability as a category of analysis akin to race, class, gender and sexuality, and a social process underlying inequality has not yet been the focus of a comprehensive and systemic historical examination.
>
> *(Gerschick and Stevens 2016 p5)*

The ASA finally introduced a section on disability a century later in 2010, although disability remains a seriously underrepresented area in relation to sociological work about inequalities (Green and Gerschick 2017). The BSA hosted the first Disability Studies Group in the same year after a comprehensive search of past and present study groups by BSA staff who expressed surprise there had been no disability group during its history [personal communication]. In the BSA, disability, if considered at all, was tucked under the umbrella of 'Medical Sociology' and treated like a reluctantly invited and lightly unruly relative at a rare family gathering. Indeed, in the executive summary of a review of 50 years of medical sociology published in the *Journal of Health and Social Behavior*, disability was mentioned in passing in one sentence (Rosich and Hankin 2010).

What is it about learning disability that is so wrong?

Civil and human rights-based calls for social justice and an end to the oppression of disabled people which emerged over 60 years ago ignored or discounted people with learning disabilities. The collective movement for social change emerging in the 1960s, was in the United States led by largely white, male, middle-class disability rights activists with considerable social capital (Berger 2019). In the United Kingdom in the main, almost completely white, largely male equivalents systematically inserted the word 'physically' in front of 'disabled' on their demands for the equal participation of disabled people. In doing so, these pioneers simply did not see or explicitly distanced themselves from people with learning disabilities, who were and remain not considered as 'disabled like me'. From the start, the slogan 'Nothing about us, without us' (Scotch 2009) adopted in countries such as the United States, Australia and the United Kingdom, was exclusionary as the movement created hierarchies of disabled identities.

The learning disability label is, furthermore, not something disabled people want attributed to them (Kittay 2001, Monteleone 2023). For example, in his memoir, disabled academic Jan Grue (2021 p46) describes being taken in a minibus to swimming rather than a gym class with his classmates.

> There were other students, too, children from the special ed classes, children who were *really* different. Not different like me; these children drooled and shouted and lashed out. Children who I could not be like, I couldn't possibly be like them, no one would think I was like them, could they? This was a new form of indignation and a new form of moral experience.

What underpins this almost visceral aversion to being considered or being associated with someone with learning disabilities is central to the disadvantages, health and wider inequalities people with learning disabilities endure. 'Learning disability' is perceived to be abhorrent while the abhorrence lies in the treatment of people so labelled.

It is instructive here to explore an example of an unusually enlightened and, at the same time, excoriating consideration of learning disabilities that pre-dates the disability movement and disability studies. *The Exoneration of the Feebleminded* was written by Kanner (1942), a psychiatrist who became better known for his work about autism. Kanner argued the dominance of the importance of cognitive ability in Western culture led to people with learning disabilities experiencing a 'double handicap' [sic] stemming from the 'type' of people they were cognitively, socially and behaviourally, and how they were perceived by others.

Kanner wrote this article after a shift in his view of people with learning disabilities because of people's participation in and contributions to the US World War Two labour. He argued the lives and opportunities of some people with learning disabilities were compromised because a focus on educational achievements does not allow consideration of contributions people can and do make. He made an explicit call for action on the part of wider society for self-education and the education of others to:

> ... extend the democratic ideal to the feebleminded, by whatever name they go, to cleanse ourselves thoroughly of the need for self-assurance by contrast, and to be friendly planners and helpers rather than carping critics and whining would-be protectors of future generations.
>
> *(Kanner 1942 p22)*

This suggestion to extend the democratic ideal to people with learning disabilities remains a contentious and anti-democratic point, as I return to later in this chapter. Kanner refers to concerns that generated well-documented eugenic practices of sterilisation to prevent the reproduction of people with learning disabilities across the United States and other countries which I return to in Chapter 2. In his plea for support and kindness, he makes a clear distinction between what he presents as a homogenous group of people with profound and multiple learning disabilities and a similarly homogenous group of people with 'milder' learning disabilities. The former comprising of people "who are not only intellectually deficient, but deficient in every sphere of mentation" (Kanner 1942 p19).

Kanner advocates for collective support for people with mild learning disabilities, writing off those he considers having no means of thinking. Around the same time, a similar proposal was enacted at the Vermont State School for Feebleminded Children (later the Brandon Training School) where children and young people with profound disabilities were warehoused while attention in the form of education and better health care, including dentistry, fresh air and nutrition, was given to those perceived to have milder learning disabilities (Allen and Fuller 2016). Kanner suggests performance is a better measure of ability than IQ tests which he likens to modified horoscope reading, to effectively release some people from the learning disability designation.

> Already many of the spastics, believed to be hopelessly inadequate until a short while ago, have been lifted out of the human waste basket and given a new lease on life and hope.
>
> *(Kanner 1942 p22)*

IQ tests have been subject to considerable critique, as Goodey (2017 p34), for example, dismisses them by illuminating the tautology that intelligence is only something measured by IQ tests, and all IQ tests do is measure intelligence. Altermark (2017) similarly describes these tests as nonsensical and unscientific. Using a Foucauldian analysis, he views the IQ test as a biopolitical tool for rule to identify failing citizens whose actions spark the need for socio-political interventions.

In some respects, whatever measure is used, a key point here is that Kanner refers to a human waste basket. Profoundly disabled people are marked as human waste, as disposable. This term is used by Razack (2021) in relation to the lives of indigenous people; disposability is a mark of sub-humanity that inscribes the lives of people who have no place in the present. The death of Jan Szamko, an asylum seeker in a detention centre in Canada, caked in faeces, is used as an example, as Razack demonstrates how disposability is a condition written on the body and amplified via Szamko's inquest where the coroner determined he died of natural causes aged 34 (Silverman and Molnar 2016). There are strong overlaps here with the lives and preventable deaths of people with learning disabilities which I return to in Chapter 2.

Of course, profoundly disabled people are not a homogenous group. The authors of a five-year Finnish study focusing on the lives of six people with profound and multiple disabilities discuss the complexity surrounding this topic in relation to one participant, Ella, who could walk (Vehmas and Mietola 2021). The authors were told by a medical professional that if a person can walk, they cannot be profoundly disabled;

> We thought Ella was especially interesting regarding our research because she challenged the conventional understanding of profound intellectual and multiple disabilities as people who lack all competence.
>
> *(Vehmas and Mietola 2021 p1)*

This statement points to wider stereotypical understandings of people with learning disabilities and the tendency of researchers to "slate over considerable differences within the group" (Altermark 2017 p20).

After a lengthy and considered period of ethnographic study, Vehmas and Mietola (2021 p177–178) conclude the lives of the people they spent time with are institutionalised with the "rhythm and content of their lives" described by support staff as narrow (kapee elämä) and shaped by basic care tasks. Ella, Anna, Hugo, Frida, Leo and Sebastian are socially isolated, buried within a disability service system designed to warehouse them, with little or no engagement with their wider community. They are in a similar position to the children at the Vermont State School, denied education, imaginaries and a life. In effect, they live ageless, non-individualised lives without any participation in everyday decisions including what or when to eat. An extended extract from the project text underlines the grimness of the findings:

> As a result, the practices and activities in group homes and day activity centres reproduced a homogenous group of people with a capacity to appreciate, generally speaking, only sensory stimuli. Care workers emphasised that many of those people who have profound intellectual disability have a capacity and desire for social interaction. However, in most group homes this desire was ignored – a circumstance that, in our view, was not only due to insufficient staff resources. Rather, it was the result of a warehousing mentality in which the threshold for an acceptable standard of care meant keeping the residents fed and clean. Everything beyond that was optional.
>
> *(Vehmas and Mietola 2021 p179)*

This warehousing is apparent in other studies of congregate care. For example, one support staff participant, Sandy, in Sirotkin's (2024 p199) study reported feeling like a 'babysitter' just there to make sure people did not hurt themselves, rather than supporting people to do things they enjoyed.

People with learning disabilities, particularly profoundly disabled people, are treated as a homogenous group by the health and social care systems, processes and practices they are enmeshed in, which are underpinned by ignorance, the paucity of, and lack of value attached to staff, and adequate support and services. Disposability inscribed on their bodies and minds allows abhorrent practices to go unchallenged. During a discussion about our *Growing Older* project findings (Ryan et al 2024a), which included people being put to bed at 5pm with the radio on, a BBC Access All Areas podcast presenter suggested that professionals listening in may say the system was working because participants had access to food and 'good lodgings'.

This presenter, and to some extent the Finnish care workers, are interpreting negative freedoms as positive attributes; freedom from hunger, poor housing and hygiene are presented as good enough or even laudable within the context of the lives of people with learning disabilities. However, as Young (2014) argues, marginalisation does not cease to be oppressive when people have food or warm shelter, and support for people with learning disabilities should mean so much more than completing tasks without deaths occuring (Capri et al 2018). Consideration of freedoms *to* participate fully in society and have meaningful lives is absent, reminding me of one Goodley's (2023 p172) provocations:

> That People with Learning Disabilities manage to exist in our communities is nothing short of astounding.

I wonder what this resilience means in practice, and how people labelled with learning disabilities deal with the intensity and depth of poor treatment – and worse – that they experience across often-shortened lifetimes. The active agency, resistance and subversiveness of people with learning disabilities is something I return to later in this chapter when discussing self-advocacy, and across this book.

More widely, however, the wider lack of interest in the lives of people with profound learning disabilities remains curious and puzzling. For Brison (2021 p118), it demonstrates "an oddly anti-intellectual attitude" for those who value intellect and suggests a "moral and epistemic failing of not caring enough to pay attention".

While I am not convinced this lack of curiosity is as benign as Brison presents, the lack of curiosity or intellectual ignorance (Goodley 2023) means there is little understanding of the lives of people with learning disabilities. The texture, colour, grimness, joy and love that characterises the everyday lives of people, their families, friends and sometimes support staff remain largely unknown. The absence of curiosity on the part of philosophers and social theorists has been described as perverse (Goodey 2017). Indeed, we seem to be stuck back with the early 20th-century sociologists who openly stood in the eugenic queue while claiming to hold the key to understanding society.

Efforts to counter these stereotypical understandings of people with profound learning disabilities include Kittay's (2020, 2009, 2002) philosophical work which draws on her experiences with her daughter Sesha, and the scholarship of de Haas (2020), whose daughter Johanna died in 2019. Both academics and mothers compellingly describe how the contributions their daughters and other people with profound learning disabilities bring need to be more widely recognised, not least in encouraging disability studies academics and activists to think more keenly about the meaning and significance of impairment.

Whether this encouragement will have much purchase within critical disability studies (Daw Srdonovic et al 2024, Garland-Thomson 2019) is unclear as scholars within this interdisciplinary field have largely ignored people with learning disabilities. Replicating the failings of the early sociologists, Garland-Thomson (2014 np) for example, describes how:

> I recognized that both framing and enacting disability in the context of the positive identity politics which emerged from the civil and human rights and social justice understanding of disability was the route to dignity, equal treatment, and access for people with disabilities.

That this route to dignity, equal treatment and access remains firmly closed to people with learning disabilities is largely overlooked within critical disability studies scholarship. Titchkosky (2003), through an analysis of Canadian 'In Unison' documents that claim to promote the integration of disabled people, describes the concept of 'able-disabled', a neoliberal and inspirational version of the person who is able conform to societal norms once physical and ideological barriers are overcome. The unwillingness to engage with or acknowledge the unable-disabled who are not able to participate 'against all the odds' creates an "ideological schism" that is ignored and yet essential to the founding premises of critical disability studies (Berger 2019 p211). The ladder to liberation from oppression has been firmly pulled up, leaving little likelihood of support for, or even engagement with, people with learning disabilities within this space. As Goodey (2017 p62) states, learning disability is not a "poor relation of physical disability within the disability category [...], rather that it is not a relation at all".

Taking a philosophical turn and considering agency

In this section, I explore how liberalism in its classic and neoliberal forms prioritises individuality, rationality and reason, of "politically sturdy citizens" who understand and fight for their rights (Abbas 2010 p40), and the consequences of this focus for people with learning disabilities. Mitchell and Snyder (2019 p194) raise the question about preferential treatment being given, even within disability academic and activist circles, to people who demonstrate an "acceptable level of resistance". There is no clear definition of what this level is or who decides it is acceptable.

Learning disability has been described as "liberalism's limit case" (Kittay 2001 p559) or a philosopher's worst nightmare (Carlson 2009). Some philosophers jostle to equate a lack of rational thinking with being less than human (see, for example, Singer 2010 and McMahan 1996), in part, to develop alternative and unconnected agendas around animal rights. As Carey (2009 p1) states,

> At no point in our history have Americans reached consensus about the extent to which people with intellectual disabilities should be allowed to exercise rights.

This is a problematic line to tread for critical disability, feminist and other theorists and it feels deeply uncomfortable that academic and intellectual tussling continues while the lives of people with learning disabilities remain largely untouched in terms of reducing oppression. Indeed, the seemingly endless creation of new and complicated terms to describe the same thing in slightly different ways acts to further distance academic, policy, social care, health and human rights discussion from the people being talked about – people who are not privy to these debates. As Mohamed (2024 p4) argues in relation to post-colonial harm in South Africa, the old problems continue and this quest to generate new epistemic terrain and different theorisations works to distract from the obvious; "Just because there are new epistemic horizons, does not mean that the world we live in has necessarily changed".

Mitchell and Snyder (2019 p194) argue for a better understanding of the lives of those who experience 'low-level agency', which they define as people who are not able to perform the role of a robust and rights-seeking citizen. The authors, drawing on their daughter's experience of intensive medical treatment involving an induced coma and nearly two years in hospital for a series of staged surgeries, (again) ask why the experience of low-level agency is not a key question in disability studies as paying attention to the experience of suffering can bring new knowledge about how to navigate such circumstances. While the suffering experienced by people with learning disabilities is typically an outcome of systemic oppression and material deprivation experienced across people's lifetimes, there is a keen absence in understanding the experience of this oppression, and a lack of interest in doing so.

These philosophical arguments have been described caustically as the 'view from nowhere' (Davy 2019) as it is unsustainable to erase the relational complexity of our everyday lives; we are all intertwined. This relationality will change over time, growing in intensity at different points and stages in our lives, shaped by our social and material situations, circumstances and intersecting identities. Being spoken on behalf of or about is something disability activists have reviled as paternalistic and a form of appropriation; however, people with learning disabilities may need to be represented by others or at least have the world around them eased in various ways to enable their space within it. This work is typically done by a group Goffman (1963) terms "the own and the wise" – in this instance, people who share or have deep knowledge and understanding of and with people with learning disabilities. *The own* are people with learning disabilities and *the wise* include family members, allies and some professionals. An exercise I undertook to crowdsource drops of brilliance from family carers (Ryan 2020) generated examples of wise professionals whose actions involved kindness, understanding, thoughtfulness, sometimes humour and care – small acts that had a considerable and long-lasting impact on family carers.

Beyond the own and the wise, health and social care professionals may not understand the consequences of their sometimes well-meaning actions in everyday life interactions. Actions which, based on ignorance about the lives, desires, aspirations and personhood of people with learning disabilities, contribute to the maintenance of structures of oppression. The work of the own and the wise in relation to people with learning disabilities typically takes place against a backdrop of a lack of knowledge, curiosity, will or ability to engage with people with learning disabilities. It is troublesome to square this ethically important representational work within disability studies and activism (Ryan and Runswick Cole 2009) where the emphasis remains on rewarding the 'doers' and 'achievers' who demonstrate independent agency (Davy 2019).

Virtually all of us will experience dependency (and caregiving) at points of our lives as we grow older, or our family members grow older or become unwell (Ward 2011). Care is an activity which links us all and was an embedded element of human societies pre-industrialisation and the advent of modernity (Jarret 2020). We need to examine these dependency relations to understand what it means to be fully human, as the concept of autonomous selfhood at the heart of the social model of disability is an illusion (Kittay 2001). For Kittay (2001), this generates a spectre where the aim is for disabled people to live their lives as non-disabled people do, again overlooking the lives of people with learning disabilities.

Binaries of dependency and autonomy, abled and non-disabled, normal and not normal are reductive and illogical. Indeed, the commitment to and almost fetishisation of rationality within liberal ideology does not hold up to scrutiny. I provide examples across this book of absurdity, deceit and the downright baffling. It is not possible to be autonomous outside of or detached from others (Goodley and Rapley 2002) as illustrated by a family friend of Kittay's daughter, Sesha:

> It's difficult to convey the delight those of us who know Sesha well take in her company. She cannot speak, let alone have a conversation or engage in witty banter. But, in her presence, one comes to realize that these things are not really necessary for communication, after all.
>
> *(Brison 2021 p103)*

The importance of supporting people to direct their own lives is prioritised and while 'agency' can be operationalised by staff and family members for people with learning disabilities (Magito McLaughlin et al 2002), this has been criticised for conflating aspects of, for example, what people are good at with what they like doing (Pilnick et al 2010), and for being the rider on which people are considered full citizens with rights (Carey 2009). Kafer (2021 p421) further critiques the neoliberal focus on aiding productivities rather than challenging systems, asking:

> What are the temporalities that unfold beyond, away from, askance of productivity, capacity, self-sufficiency, independence, achievement?

The prioritisation of agency over-privileges the role of autonomy, rationality and choice as determinants of what constitutes a good life. A focus that allows an avoidance of responsibility, of the necessary work, for really thinking about what makes a good life (Reinders 2000). Disentangling the complex strands that weave through people's lives is troublesome, and considering a partial and shifting focus on autonomy, rationality and choice generates discomfort and incomprehension. The overwhelming strength of normative expectations and determined resistance to recognising what people with learning disabilities contribute, leaves understandings of the lives of people with learning disabilities compromised and allows space for assumptions and ignorance to thrive. It seems odd to still be puzzling over basic questions about citizenship and what constitutes a good life a quarter of the way through the 21st century. We have a social model of disability showing us how *not* to lead disabled lives, and people with learning disabilities expected to demonstrate agency without any real sense for who. Carey (2009 p219) calls this controlled integration; people with learning disabilities are effectively situated in spaces that demand conformity or, in the case of intimate lives, as I explore in Chapter 4, erasure.

For Carey (2009), there has been a focus in academia on the idea that people with learning disabilities are different from other people and their exclusion rests in their 'condition', or the social construction of the condition. This is difficult to accept however, when thinking about, for example, the forensic examination of the 'In Unison' documents discussed earlier based on an excoriating take of disability mattering as a problem-of-exclusion (Titchkosky 2003 p518). How can critical disability scholars, with few exceptions, ignore this thing called learning disability?

Rights for people with learning disabilities are positioned within a relational cost–benefit analysis which involves thinking about the potentially negative consequences for other citizens and social institutions (Carey 2009). This is clearly illustrated in Chapter 3 when I discuss enduring fears around reproduction and eugenic practices. The acceptance of socially constructed difference and exclusion on the part of academics is also evidenced in the *ASA Status Committee on Persons with Disability in Sociology* report (Green and Gerschick 2017) which found sociological articles about disability in the United States are almost all published in the *Journal of Health and Social Behaviour*.

If we move beyond these established conventions of agency, we start to see examples of reciprocity, activism and subversiveness that are commonly overlooked, or ignored. These include the actions of young people at the Brandon Training School, where examples of survival, noncompliance, pleasure-seeking and gestural and emotional expression were identified among the residents (Allen and Fuller 2016). Indeed, these authors suggest we might learn from looking at the history of one of Canada's large institutions to question a liberal, rights-based model of disability justice which will always leave some people out. Examples of love, kindness and care apparent among inmates are salutary in the face of what were (and sometimes continue to be) systems of neglect, abuse and brutality. The importance of reciprocity in living a good life was also apparent in our *Flourishing Lives* project (Ryan and O'Brien 2024). Giving, on a grand scale or lifting someone's day with a smile, is core to being human, yet is all too often discounted or ignored.

The outcome of these enduring and apparently irresolvable discussions around who counts as a citizen is that people with learning disabilities live what have been described as 'non-livable' lives (Taylor 2013). This creates conditions for foreseeable, avoidable and acceptable ill treatment, physical violence and harm, bringing us back to social murder.

> Where lives are unrecognized, individuals become exposed to physical violence precisely because that physical violence is not at present recognized as harm. Their pain, their loss, is un-grievable.
>
> *(Taylor 2013 np)*

Johnson (2018 p134, drawing on Durkheim 1898/1969) highlights the absence of collective respect for the empty space around *all* our bodies which is the basis of a humane and kind society. This not only allows but also facilitates certain people to be considered "good to mistreat" (Hughes 2019 p830). Numerous, countless even, examples of state sanctioned violence against and harm of people with learning disabilities in the United Kingdom and wider exist. A review of 26 of the 77 people with learning disabilities and/or autistic people living in long-term segregation in hospital units in England found one person waited 19 years to be discharged and several people gained criminal records while inpatients (Hollins 2023). These details can overwhelm and cancel themselves out, not least because benchmarks are absent in these abhorrent landscapes. We do not know how many patients gain criminal records as NHS inpatients. While nearly half the units attempted to make segregation rooms more 'homelike', the remainder ranged from single rooms to high security environments which included empty cells with hatches for surveillance, communication and to deliver meals. Hollins (2023) concluded:

> The humanity of people in solitary confinement gets forgotten. Their life story remains unknown. The use of solitary confinement affects the person's identity to such an extent it causes what could be described as a 'social death'.

It is not a leap to link consideration of social murder to the experiences of people with learning disabilities incarcerated in segregated settings or solitary confinement in the United Kingdom, to the language of spectres, hauntings and half-lives used in post-institutionalisation scholarship. As Series (2022 p11) argues, the care world operates in a different legal space where people become "legal ghosts; half there, half not".

The UK government rebutted most of the 12 recommendations of the Hollins report which included providing access to independent advocacy, specialist free legal advice and the use of solitary confinement to be included in the category of "never events" for children and young people under 18 (Gov UK 2023). These recommendations aimed to empower people with learning disabilities, autistic people and family members through legal and human rights-based support and strengthen the role of the state in the scrutiny of people incarcerated in these units. The report was commissioned in response to well-publicised concerns about lengthy stays and difficulties in discharging people from these units. The lack of subsequent action or even interest generated by the report provides further evidence of the acceptance of non-livable lives and the associated mistreatment of people with learning disabilities.

The Hollins report provides clear and contemporary evidence of the conditions for social murder and the refusal of the government to act on these. Casual reference to solitary confinement in relation to people with learning disabilities (who have committed no crime) is extraordinary when considered alongside the weight of evidence in the criminology field where solitary confinement in prisons is perceived to be the most punitive and dangerous intervention alongside the death penalty (Sobel and Smith 2019).

There is no such consideration for people incarcerated in these so-called assessment and treatment units. Indeed, a group of psychiatrists published a critique of Hollins' report condoning the use of long-term segregation (Tromans et al 2024). Their arguments can be summarised as: segregation can be more acceptable than forced medication and restraint, some autistic people may choose to be alone because of sensory issues and psychiatrists know best. A concluding sentence highlights the defensiveness of their response as they argue care of the vulnerable should be "underpinned by evidence-based medicine and not ideologically driven opinion" (Tromans et al 2024 np).

In the United Kingdom, after Baroness Hale's ruling in the case of *P v Cheshire West and Chester Council and another*, it is recognised that people who have been released from institutionalisation can also be deprived of their liberty in their own homes leading to the emergence of contested and liminal care spaces that have similar characteristics to institutions (Series 2022 p5).

The continuation of abuse in congregate and supported living settings is chilling. That support staff are trained how to restrain people generates an expectation of the need for restraint and staff can be recruited with restraint in mind. Support staff have described how anyone can be recruited and could be "itching for a fight" (Sirotkin 2024). When considering the powerlessness of people with learning disabilities in these often-closed settings, this is a deeply concerning reflection. Sirotkin (2024) further found staff would excuse and not report abusive actions on the part of colleagues, rationalising their action as not "crossing the line" because the actions of the person being supported warranted intervention or the potential repercussions for the reported staff member could be serious. It was also difficult to evidence harms witnessed which led to a lack of safeguarding action. Inaction is seen as more acceptable than intervention, systemic neglect is normalised and violence justified.

It feels strikingly naive now to reflect on what we know about post-institutionalisation, and the uncritical optimism that closing institutions and moving people back into communities would somehow magic away the systematic discounting of people with learning disabilities. Post-institutionalisation has not involved a shift of power from government to people with learning disabilities; instead, control has changed in form to crafting citizens, surveillance and managing conduct by brute force where necessary (Altermark 2017 p4). Part of the problem is the widespread absorption and circulation of a narrative of gradual progression from pre- to post-institutionalisation which acts to conceal the rule of the present.

> The era of post-institutionalisation testifies to precisely this – how something that we in hindsight easily detect as horrendous can give way to something else, a new mode of governing which continues to constrain the lives of people with intellectual disabilities but which we all too easily fail to acknowledge.
>
> *(Altermark 2017 p157)*

The number of people who remain incarcerated in assessment and treatment units in the United Kingdom, currently estimated at 2185 (Glasby et al 2024), despite numerous national initiatives since the Winterbourne View scandal in 2011, speaks to this brute force. Contradiction is at the heart of the rhetoric around inclusion, autonomy and independence, and how people who form the otherness category in relation to these ideals can possibly be considered citizens. Turning again to Altermark (2017), there is a haunting of what is always excluded to present a reasonable characterisation of humanity.

Two further examples are useful here to illustrate the contradictions and precarious position or even existence of people with learning disabilities. Carey (2009) highlights a class action suit on behalf of all retarded [sic] children excluded from education in 1972 – the Pennsylvania Association for Retarded Children *Parc v Pennsylvania*. The outcome of this class action was, or should have been, important in reconceptualising the basis of granting rights in the United States as Justice Thomas Masterson's enlightened opinion was based on a position that all children have the potential to benefit from education. His underlying principle was that people receive rights because they *are* citizens, rather than based on criteria such as reason or cognition.

A little more than a decade later, Cleburne City denied a developer permission to convert a building into independent supported flats for 13 people with learning disabilities. This decision was upheld by the Supreme Court in *City of Cleburne, Texas vs Cleburne Living Center* (1985). The Supreme Court supported the argument made by Cleburne City that the proposal was for a "hospital for the feebleminded" which needed a special permit. Gaps in the Supreme Court judgement included no challenge around calling these homes a hospital and the city was not required to justify its arguments. Carey (2009) raises contradictions that still exist in that while there may be national support for the legal equality of people with learning disabilities, fears remain around the operationalisation of this support in terms of the best interests of people with learning disabilities and the communities in which they live. The Cleburne City example speaks to the prioritisation of the rights of non-disabled people and children to lead their lives unsullied by the presence of people with learning disabilities. One of the arguments against the supported flats in Cleburne, for example, was the potential the development had for decreasing the serenity and safety of the neighbourhood. While the court found Cleburne City had been discriminatory due to fears of learning disability, it failed to define people with learning disabilities as a "suspect class" which would have offered future protections.

Taylor (2013) suggests we should ask if philosophical questions about life and moral status work to distort alternative conceptions of competency, ability and well-being *in advance* of questions about human life and moral status. What is hidden by this consistent focus on agency, rationality and reasoning? Taylor (2013) argues we should address the social conditions under which qualifiers for moral status and human belonging arise and ask what the qualifying conditions are for both. Arguments about demarcating lines and newly formed norms reinforce the trope of 'liveable lives', that is, lives that count whereas all lives count. We all matter. These philosophical questions and discussions position the humanity of people with learning disabilities as somehow 'suspect' (without suspect class protections) whereas philosophers should revise their conceptions of personhood, so their theories include everyone (Wong 2007).

Philosophical debate objectifies, alienates and disenfranchises disabled people, in particular people with learning disabilities (Monteleone 2024). We need to reimagine what is philosophical and wider knowledge and knowledge makers, not least because people with learning disabilities and other marginalised groups have not been included in these debates about their lives and their personhood, and on this note I turn to consider self-advocacy.

Self-advocacy

The civil rights movement of self-advocacy among people with learning disabilities has a history as long as, albeit on a smaller scale, the early physical disability rights activists discussed above. The first meeting of self-advocates was held in England in 1972 and the first People First International conference in Washington State, USA, in 1984 (Walmsley 2022).

There is a tension between individual confidence building and collective campaigning in this movement, although self-advocacy can be the basis for "subtle radicalism" supporting political agency *and* self-confidence (Anderson and Bigby 2017). Self-advocacy programmes and involvement are empowering (Chong et al 2024, Krueger et al 2024, Mineur et al 2017), and involve positive freedoms such as learning new skills, acquiring new knowledge, extending social relationships, providing employment opportunities and support to change personal circumstances such as housing (Tilley et al 2020). For example, one participant in an Australian study described how,

> ... since I've come into this group I've been part of the group, I feel loved and cared for and everyone here is so nice and caring and friendly, and they're always here for me, so I'm glad I'm here with you guys.
>
> *(Strnadová et al 2018, p1096)*

Self-advocacy offers opportunities and freedoms to develop different identities (Anderson and Bigby 2015). Groups are, however, seriously hindered by a lack of funding and resources for organising support staff, transport and meetings (Petri et al 2021), and the involvement of profoundly disabled people has not materialised. The poor historical documenting of the English self-advocacy movement has been attributed in part due to a struggle to survive (Walmsley 2022), while large charities that claim to fight for human rights and equality, such as Mencap in England, can maintain or contribute to inequalities (Petri et al 2021).

People remain, instead, largely epistemically oppressed and prevented from contributing to knowledge production. These clear injustices strongly point to structural prejudice and ignorance about the lives and experiences of people with learning disabilities and bring me to discuss some approaches I draw upon across this book.

Epistemic injustice and inclusion phobia

Discussion about agency, rationality and reason, and arguments about whether people qualify as citizens, or are somehow less than or non-human, revolve around knowledge and knowing. Who knows what, and how do we know this? Who has the power to dictate, legitimate or dismiss what constitutes knowledge? As people with learning disabilities are largely excluded from these discussions, which are typically conducted using tangled, academic, technical and complicated language, little is known about what people know, and how they feel about and experience their lives and the lives of those around them.

Fricker's (2007) concept of epistemic injustice involves knowledge, understanding, power and obstruction. She identifies two types of epistemic injustice: testimonial injustice which involves people being disbelieved or discounted because of who they are, and hermeneutical injustice which refers to gaps in collective (and accessible) resources which puts people at a disadvantage in terms of making sense of their experiences (Fricker 2007 p1). People with learning disabilities are clearly disadvantaged in terms of sense-making because of the lack of accessible information, support and resources. There are also wider gaps in the collective resources, around what we know about certain issues, which lead to misinterpretations and the dominance of largely negative assumptions. Practices of segregation can further fuel hermeneutical injustice as commentary around not knowing how to engage with people with learning disabilities continues today. One example of a comment from a social work student during a seminar held while writing this book; "I don't know any people with learning disabilities, I don't know how to talk to them".

Hermeneutical injustice is structural, a product of social powerlessness as people are marginalised from meaning-making activities (Anderson 2012) and the role of epistemic agency of privileged groups and individuals is key in its production and reproduction (Pohlhaus 2012). For Fricker (2007), testimonial injustice cuts deeply as it involves being excluded from the practice of what it is to know. We have already seen how people with learning disabilities are excluded from discussion about their personhood. They are further effectively excluded from being a "knower" which means they are unable to develop as epistemic subjects (Dohmen 2016), although a strength of the self-advocacy movement is generating opportunities for people to develop knowledge about their rights, and their lives (Tilley 2022). The wrongs for people with learning disabilities cut particularly deep because, as we have seen, there is little evidence their lives and aspirations matter. Being excluded from being a "knower" can lead to experiences of harm and abuse continuing unchecked, effectively allowing the denial of personhood.

Learning disability complicates this focus on knowledge and knowing as the focus prioritises reason and rationality. However, being discounted and the associated lack of understanding around the lives of people with learning disabilities is a key part of the continuing oppression. Even if people try to convey their experiences (and they may not be able to do so because of the lack of epistemic resources), they are not listened to because of this lack of understanding. That is, hermeneutical injustice feeds testimonial injustice because of a lack of possible sense-making (Kalman et al 2016).

An example of testimonial injustice was provided by Marie Sepulchre in her keynote presentation at the Disability Studies conference held at Leeds University, United Kingdom, in September 2024. She described a growing friendship with a 60-year-old Belgian man with learning disabilities who wanted to write an autobiography. Struck by his insights into his own life and wider society, she worked with him to write the book and offered some of these insights as part of her presentation. The man's sister, however, was alarmed by the project and after reading the draft version of the book, said her brother would not speak or think like that. The book project was shelved as the man did not want conflict with his sister who was also his legal guardian. The sister arguably exercised her epistemic power, preventing her brother from contributing his knowledge of his life and experiences.

Not knowing is a form of ignorance, and a key question is what motivates epistemic ignorance on the part of those who have the social capital and power to know and yet choose not to. As Alcoff (2007) describes, ignorance is not simply a lack of knowledge; it is a substantial epistemic practice that demands examination. How far is ignorance wilful as dominant groups refuse to become proficient in the epistemic resources necessary to attend to these absences? The term 'scholarship of the obvious' has been introduced to underline how normalised and ordinary overlooked scandals and violences are (Mohamed 2024). Dotson (2012 p32) suggests a form of wilful hermeneutical ignorance which continues when the hearer refuses to be more open. Indeed, it has been suggested that new skills and patience will be needed from those who typically discredit, silence or deny the knowledge of people with learning disabilities (Dohmen 2016 p682).

I am reminded of Eva Kittay's (2009) attempt while at a conference with fellow philosopher Peter Singer to persuade him to take a short journey to visit the group home where her daughter Sesha lived. Singer, who has strong beliefs that non-human animals and profoundly disabled people are morally on a par, refused, asking what he would see that would change his argument. Kittay, in thinking about this refusal and their exchanges during the conference, later reflected how:

> What is especially salient in all our exchanges is that in all their writings about people with significant cognitive impairments, philosophers like Singer and

> McMahan presume to know the capabilities of the people they write about when, as I have attempted to demonstrate, they know virtually nothing at all.
> *(Kittay 2009 p618)*

Kittay calls for epistemic modesty, and the importance of taking concrete steps to know what we do not know. However, the wilfully ignorant are too often motivated not to acknowledge what they should know. In her research into the review of the abuse at mother and baby homes in Ireland in the last century, O'Donnell (2023 p233), introduces the term 'belligerent ignorance' to describe an active resistance to engaging with countervailing information, evidence, arguments or even apparent appeals to legal or moral norms.

Wilful or belligerent ignorance can be a mechanism to silence marginalised groups, facilitating the production and reproduction of class, ableist, gender and racist hierarchies. For example, a 'banal' technique of neglect is diversion where people are obstructed from understanding their rights and eligibility for local authority services by professionals maintaining "a constructive opacity around eligibility requirements" (Keily and Warnock 2023 p329). People can be forced to spend time trying to understand what information they need to provide to access support, thereby slowing the flow of cases into overstretched services. This deliberate and wilful technique of obfuscation again cuts deeper for people with learning disabilities who are already disadvantaged within this space because of the lack of accessible information and support.

Marginalised groups can, of course, develop their own resources as a form of resistance or have epistemic resources which are simply not recognised as such (Kalman et al 2016). We neglect essential, embodied knowledge because it is not articulated in spoken or written words which are prized as credible. Arguably, *the wise,* as illustrated by the extract from Brison earlier talking about the delight she experienced in Sesha's company, recognise and engage with these epistemic resources. They may be unable, however, to support the acceptance of this knowledge into collective epistemic resources, which is the wider set of knowledge we share and draw upon in our everyday lives.

Testimonial injustice can be eased by ensuring equitable participation, listening to people and taking them seriously. Hermeneutical injustice is more challenging to resolve as a significant area of experience is obscured from collective understanding (Dotson 2014). Ideas of what would be epistemically just in interactions with people with learning disabilities, particularly people with profound learning disabilities include being open to and taking seriously expressions of pleasure, pain, likes and dislikes of people, or those close to them (Dohmen 2016). This is, in effect, an expression of decency and respectfulness that draws me again to Durkheim's concept of moral individualism which he argues concerns people in general rather than individuals; respect, compassion and care for people is the by-product of the collective belief in the sacredness of everyone (Johnson 2018). In Chapter 2, I draw on the concept of narrative humility (DasGupta 2008) which, similarly, involves health professionals listening to patients and trying to fully understand people's experiences.

Sadly, there is little evidence that suggests those who discredit, deny or silence people with learning disabilities, or family carers, are open to developing different ways of knowing or doing, and reform of current unjust institutions seems unlikely. The term 'epistemically vulnerabised' has been used to refer to people "whose epistemic dice are already loaded against them" because of their backgrounds and identities (Carel and Kidd 2021 p475). There are, however, glimmers of light. For example, Altermark (2017 p139) writes about the group interview he held with Swedish self-advocates who unexpectedly forced him to learn how to listen, thereby demonstrating to him the importance of resistance as forcing people to "unlearn their inability to acknowledge the viewpoints of people with intellectual disabilities".

Another perspective I consider is Goodey's (2017) articulation of inclusion phobia. Goodey explicitly steers clear of ethical or moral reflections in arguing that learning disability is the product of a more general inclusion phobia where the tendency for societies to establish an ingroup and inevitable outgroups reaches an extreme point. Goodey argues our attention should focus on this phobia rather than people labelled with learning disabilities.

He describes how the concept of learning disability shifts with different iterations, labels and definitions over time. While the label disappears the further we go back in time, the clearer it is defined, the more inevitable the segregating practices that go with it. He again highlights the blanket omission of learning disability in the theorising of so many scholars, even those focusing on the dehumanisation of marginalised groups, referencing Douglas (1966), Tajfel (1981) and Rachman (2004), among others. Just as learning disability is liberalism's limit, it is an exemplar of inclusion phobia and there is little or no curiosity about why people may be phobic. Goodey's concept of inclusion phobia allows us to see how people with learning disabilities are subject to mistreatment and health inequalities with apparent disinterest from wider society.

Discussion in this chapter and the wider work upon which it is based, speaks to a clear and urgent need for change, for dismantling systems of oppression that deny the humanity of certain groups of people who seemingly have no place in the present. As Altermark (2017) suggests, we need to develop a language and terminology that does not take for granted ideals, such as independence or agency that the politics of inclusion are based on. We need to view these concepts as shrouding discourses that make possible only certain ways of doing and thinking. We could interpret this gap in language and terminology as a form of hermeneutical injustice, one that is supported by many who should know better and do differently. Across this book, I provide examples of these injustices and hope the reader is able to develop a better understanding of the violences people with learning disabilities experience which are too often overlooked or seen as natural as the air around us.

What is your relationship to disability?

I have felt considerable discomfort writing this book, in particular the ethical implications of writing about people with learning disabilities which includes speaking for (not about) people rather than with them (Goodley 2023). O'Toole (2013) offers what has been described as a disability identity best practice 'outing' plan (Garland-Thomson 2014) which involves non-disabled people who engage in disability matters answering the question 'What is your relationship to disability?' While O'Toole presents a set of potential categories such as disabled person, parent, ally, sister, which could be included in brackets after people's names, her question also opens opportunities for storytelling.

My beautiful son Connor, who died a throwaway and preventable death aged 18 (Ryan 2017) is the heart, the kick starter and underlying commitment to my relationships, as a mother, friend, scholar activist and colleague, to disability. My intertwined, interwoven relationships with people with learning disabilities and family carers in personal, activist and academic spaces bring consistent warmth, love, joy and critical challenge.

Altermark (2017) underlines the importance of creating spaces for politicisation and to consistently challenge assumptions about the limitations of people with learning disabilities. I suggest focusing our attention on challenging these assumptions is misplaced, sucking us back into debates prioritising agency, rationality and autonomy. We should, as Goodey (2017) argues, focus on the conditions that generate inclusion phobia and the actions that support it.

I discussed earlier suggestions to generate hermeneutical and testimonial justice by listening to and treating people with respect, trying to understand their lives and experiences. While our social reality is made up of interdependence, interconnection and encounters, we too often do not have the social imagination to recognise this. Braidotti (2012) argues for an elaboration of what it is to live joyfully and not be drawn by negative judgements. Other scholars, similarly, try to identify ways of breaking out of the "socially perpetuated straitjackets of constraint, limit or coercion" (Mitchell and Snyder 2019 p189) and avoid the negativity much scholarship produces. Garland-Thomson reminds us of stories of disability as occasions for human flourishing, of wonder and transformation. She further advocates seeking reparative readings of disability which "recognise resourcefulness, creativity and persistence – the persistence of disability in the world and those who inhabit it" (Garland-Thomson 2014 np). Throughout this book I include examples of the persistence, resourcefulness and creativity of people with learning disabilities. This is not to objectify or tokenise these experiences, instead to highlight that which is often overlooked or discounted.

Book structure

This book is divided into five chapters which loosely follow key social determinants of health and well-being. My commitment to following these determinants lessened over time as the more I read, the more the inconsistencies and contradictions, and the distorting or breaking of rules, processes and contexts with the underlining aim to constrain the lives of people with learning disabilities, became apparent. Health inequalities, while of course relevant to people with learning disabilities, are not necessarily a defining contributor to people's lives, health and wellbeing. Indeed, as we see throughout the book social determinants of health may not have the same impact they have on people without learning disabilities.

In Chapter 2, I discuss timely and effective access to healthcare and focus upon key interventions and areas including annual health checks, diagnostic overshadowing, preventable deaths and inadequate investigatory processes. These areas raise troubling practices and evidence of social murder which include wilful ignorance around processes, a lack of confidence or knowledge about treating people labelled with learning disabilities and discounting premature deaths. The chapter ends with discussion of the role of the research community in contributing to oppressive practices. During the process of writing this book, the substance of the failings of the research community has grown in magnitude, if not intent.

Chapter 3 focuses on sexual intimacy and relationships and documents how national eugenic programmes have been replaced with less explicit forms of eugenics which include surveillance, arbitrary provider rules and a lack of support and accessible information to enable people to develop intimate relationships. I discuss the ways in which systems of protection are misused to prevent sexual relationships, pregnancy and parenting, and demonstrate how absurdities creep into this area as sexuality, intimacy and pregnancy generate documented and extreme phobic responses from a range of people and professionals.

In Chapter 4, I explore aspects of housing, including affordability, quality and neighbourhood, and employment. This chapter again draws on international research to demonstrate similarities in experiences and identifiable mechanisms of obstruction to a good life. Employment, as a key determinant of health, was originally planned to be a stand-alone chapter; however, it became apparent that while much is researched and written about this area, there has been a risible impact on the lives of people with learning disabilities. I am not condoning this position, I simply want to avoid adding to white noise in this area by writing into it listing empty recommendations and failed interventions.

In Chapter 5, I use eating and food practices as an exemplar to pull together and further develop or provide substance to key arguments developed across the book. Eating is as universal as falling in love and sleeping, and yet for people labelled with learning disabilities, it is often a further site of constraint, dismissal and sometimes neglect and harm. I discuss the findings of the *Flourishing Lives* project which introduce some sense and light in this area, before moving on to a postscript summarising the key insights and arguments generated by this journey across the landscape of learning disability related research, nearly a quarter of the way through the 21st century.

2

ACCESSING HEALTHCARE

Introduction

While the World Health Organisation (WHO) stipulates the importance of affordable access to healthcare of a decent quality, the public health systematic review evidence base is weak and uneven in terms of what interventions work in tackling social determinants of health (Bambra et al 2010). Existing evidence also features little consideration of the experiences of people with learning disabilities in the Global South (Robertson et al 2019). Evidence that exists highlights the problems, limitations, drawbacks and systemic failures that surround access to healthcare for people with learning disabilities. It is not possible to consider much of this scholarship here or sensible to try given the often lacklustre impact it has on the health and wellbeing of people with learning disabilities. Instead, I focus on key areas of annual health checks, 'diagnostic overshadowing', mortality rates, death investigations and how the academic community through its research and reporting practices contributes to the epistemic injustices people experience. The first four areas provide insights into enduring issues, contradictions and failings, and provide a clear, health-related trail to the social murder of people with learning disabilities. The fifth area, which could have been included within any chapter, intends to remind researchers we should work from a place of acknowledging the potential we all have to be oppressive or harmful (Sirotkin 2024 p279).

A longstanding resistance to considering social inequalities and wider systemic issues around mechanisms of power and subordination means health is often viewed as an individual issue (Hill 2015). The problem lies within the person and they are to blame for challenges they may face. We clearly see this in operation under the current Labour government whose manifesto includes an emphasis on 'working people' and there are targeted attacks on 'work-shy' people in receipt of

DOI: 10.4324/9781032644868-2

benefits. There is little or no acknowledgement or recognition of enduring systemic and structural inequalities which leave the health needs of marginalised people, including people with learning disabilities, compromised, ignored or deliberately targeted. Popay (2010) argued over a decade ago that health inequalities will not lessen until the public health community recognise these as an issue of social injustice and publicly speak up. This has not happened despite the explicit responsibility of medical professionals to oppose, individually and collectively, the forces that contribute to health inequalities (Donohoe 2012, p602).

A direct call to the nursing profession to not be moral bystanders, to not, intentionally or unintentionally, remain silent in the face of injustice has similarly been largely ignored (McGibbon and Lukeman 2019). These authors characterise moral bystanding as a foundational barrier to critical action, and an act of violence. It should not be a feature of health and social care practice and yet remains resolutely intact and evidenced across different areas of, for example, the NHS in the United Kingdom, including learning disability, maternity and mental health services (Goodwin 2019). Young (2014) refers to the sometimes unconscious assumptions and reactions of 'well-meaning' people in everyday life; however, this interpretation downgrades the impact of these reactions. An integral part of the work of health and social care professionals should involve knowing and engaging with what DasGupta (2008) in a medical context describes as narrative humility. That is, careful, kind and attentive listening to patients to understand the context of their lives as fully as possible. This articulation of narrative humility is relevant to everyone and, as mentioned in Chapter 1, is about the open space around us all. It should not be considered a particular technique or intervention for engaging with certain patient groups. Indeed, DasGupta (2008 p981) reminds us how all stories have elements of the unfamiliar, not just the stories of those who may be perceived as 'other'; within the clinical relationship "the clinician must not only see, but be seen, and by doing so, enable herself to see even more clearly".

DasGupta further highlights the importance of *kind knowing* as a professional. There are no excuses for not knowing and yet we have health and social care systems in which professionals too often demonstrate ignorance and associated cruelty. Moral courage is needed, the antecedents of which are conscience and ethical sensitivity (McGibbon and Lukeman 2019). Moral courage, however, has been appropriated and diluted by, for example, the language of whistleblowing in various countries, including the United Kingdom, USA and Canada with associated deadening policies, processes and protections (see, for example, Ash 2016). As a good friend, who was a health visitor, some decades ago commented, "We didn't used to whistleblow, we just said when something was wrong". For Sirotkin (2024), while whistleblowing policies do not work or offer protections, the assumptions underpinning whistleblowing procedures, including the legal and regulatory frameworks that surround them, limit our ability to respond to wrongs. There is an assumption that safeguarding interventions apply to exceptional circumstances which reduces responsibility to attend to harms witnessed, thereby reducing the likelihood of saying when something is *wrong*. As we will repeatedly see across this book, the processes designed to protect people and support them to raise concerns do not work.

With this in mind, and building on discussion from Chapter 1, here I focus on epistemic ignorance, on what people know and do not act on, on what people do not know and should know and what people refuse to know. McGibbon and Lukeman (2019) include the intentional and unintentional in their articulation of moral bystanding. This aligns with epistemic ignorance as not knowing and wilful ignorance as an act of refusing to know. For trained professionals, not knowing in the sense of being unaware is not acceptable practice. Working on the basis of unconscious assumptions and being well-meaning is simply not good enough. The individualisation of health, coupled with the often ignorant, discriminatory and prejudicial views of health and social care professionals, reflected in wider society, contribute to persistent inequalities around accessing appropriate and effective healthcare, and the subsequent preventable deaths of people with learning disabilities.

The stark health care rationing and treatment of disabled people globally during the COVID-19 pandemic is a powerful example of this. An international scoping review found disabled people, including people with learning disabilities, were excluded from services including intensive care beds and lifesaving equipment and subjected to Do Not Attempt Cardiopulmonary Resuscitation (DNACPR) notices with no discussion with the person, their family members or support workers (Taggart et al 2022). People from ethnic minority groups faced worse outcomes (Hassiotis 2020). These notices were not conjured out of air, they were decided upon and applied by health professionals, unchallenged by other health and social care staff.

The consequences were harrowing. In the first year of the pandemic, COVID-19 was the leading cause of death among people with learning disabilities in the United States, compared to the third leading cause of death for the wider population (Landes et al 2022). State-level rationing algorithms were exposed (Lund and Ayres 2020) and in some states, state-level crisis standards of care included categorical exclusions around impairments (Chicoine et al 2022). In Ontario, Canada, people with learning disabilities were two times more likely to be hospitalised with COVID-19 and to die from it than the general population (Lunsky et al 2022). In the United Kingdom, people with learning disabilities were four times more likely to be hospitalised than non-disabled people with a tenfold risk of death among patients with Down Syndrome (Clift et al 2021, Flynn et al 2021, Flynn et al 2022). Once hospitalised, people with learning disabilities had a 56% increased risk of death and died 1.44 times faster than other patients (Baksh et al 2021).

This is a clear example of social murder globally and while the slow wheels of public inquiry are turning in some countries, for example, England, there have been few or no consequences or apparent reflections by those who made these decisions. I suspect adherence to this rationing is still seen as appropriate by many.

Neglected treatment needs or treated differently?

People with learning disabilities often do not receive appropriate or timely healthcare. The list of absences in people's healthcare experiences is lengthy and comprehensively researched. Absent are: responsive services; sufficient assessment; knowledge; sense; uptake of preventative healthcare and screening; care; monitoring and treatment of chronic conditions; early cancer detection; accessible communication and information; and consistent understandings of mental capacity. Filling these absences are (again) assumptions which work as the basis upon which healthcare is often delivered. These include the view that people with learning disabilities are inherently unhealthy and/or do not matter and are people who lack capacity to engage with their own healthcare; and prejudice, awkwardness and embarrassment among staff and the ever-present ignorance (see, for example, Anderson et al 2013, Appelgren et al 2018, Cuypers et al 2022, Guttman et al 2021, Pelleboer-Gunnink et al 2017).

Clinical guidelines, viewed as a staple of robust healthcare through the systematic evaluation of the evidence base and contribution to cost-effective healthcare, could be used to address health inequalities. However, concern has been raised that guidelines can increase health inequalities by potentially improving the health of those with existing health advantages. A review of guidelines from seven countries found most did not contain content relevant to people with learning disabilities or identify they may be at increased risk of certain health issues (Mizen et al 2012).

This evidence leads me to argue people with learning disabilities do not have 'neglected' treatment needs, they are instead treated differently to other patients. They are an outgroup of patients often excluded from consideration of narrative humility. I am not sure people with learning disabilities even qualify as 'patients' as treatment can be lacking in the most basic care. Reading literature in this area is uncomfortable because of similarities in research findings and recommendations in different parts of the world and over time, none of which are groundbreaking or necessarily difficult or costly to achieve. I provide some examples of this work here to illustrate well-trodden issues in terms of research focus, findings and recommendations.

Research involving people with learning disabilities demonstrates how they can be fearful of receiving bad news, struggle to understand inaccessible communication or feel unable to express how they are feeling to health professionals (Tilly 2013). Recommendations included better identification of patients with learning disabilities, better use of tablet dispenser dosage packs and accessible communications.

A study involving five people with learning disabilities and family carers had more innovative findings alongside the importance of accessible communications. Participants underlined the importance of touch and of staff acting less professionally. For example, one family carer described how:

> James had an IV [intravenous] thingy in, he didn't really like it, so the surgeon just kind of pulled it out and said 'goodbye' and threw it away [laughs] and the nurses were tutting, because it meant there was like a needle on the floor somewhere, but he just instantly got it.
>
> *(Badcock and Sakellariou 2022 np)*

A systematic review of professional attitudes about learning disability (with the caveat that many of the 30 papers included from nine countries, including India, New Zealand, United Kingdom, the United States and Israel, were designated not good quality), found professionals were ignorant about learning disability and people were seen as different, as "childlike, funny, strange or intimidating" (Pelleboer-Gunninket et al 2017 p431). The study concluded health professionals need learning disability awareness training involving people with learning disabilities, and that research needs to move beyond descriptions of stigma.

A systematic review focused on nursing in eight countries describes the lack of awareness among registered nurses as a "breeding ground" for othering patients with learning disabilities (Appelgren et al 2018). An international integrative review of literature about access to healthcare between 2001 and 2018 found training, knowledge and awareness, communication, fear and embarrassment, lack of involvement in healthcare decision making and time were barriers to accessing primary care for people with learning disabilities (Doherty et al 2020).

In the United Kingdom, repeated recommendations include training healthcare professionals and awareness raising. In a country with over 80 years of universal healthcare access 'free to all at the point of delivery', it seems anomalous to acknowledge that training needs around providing healthcare for certain patient groups remain outstanding. Having undergone years of medical education and training, health professionals are ill-equipped to engage with patients with learning disabilities. This is despite widespread knowledge of the well-documented health inequalities and shortened lives people with learning disabilities experience. I can assert this is widespread knowledge because it is unfathomable that UK-based health and social care professionals cannot know given a series of high-profile scandals that stretch back across decades and include Ely hospital (Butler and Drakeford 2005), Winterbourne View (Flynn and Citarella 2013) and Whorlton Hall (Hough 2023).

There is some contradiction in evidence about the prevalence of long-term conditions and ill health among people with learning disabilities. For example, death from cancer has been reported as 1.5 times more likely in people with learning disabilities in the Netherlands (Cuypers et al 2022) and a Swedish population-based cohort study found a 1.6-fold increase in cancer risk in people with learning disabilities (up to the age of 43), with an increased cancer risk for several types of cancer, including colon, pancreas and kidney (Liu et al 2021). A second Swedish study found people with learning disabilities aged 55 and over had a lower cancer rate than the general population (Satgé et al 2020). Other studies have found lower or similar rates of cancer among people with learning disabilities and the mainstream population. Carey et al (2017) found people with learning disabilities have lower recording of cancer and coronary heart disease than the general population although greater levels of chronic disease.

These disparities may be accounted for by lifestyle factors or inequalities in screening and cancer care for people with learning disabilities. For example, evidence suggests people with learning disabilities with cancer are likely to be diagnosed in an emergency and with a later stage cancer. Delayed cancer diagnoses in the United Kingdom have been attributed to a lack of awareness about how cancer presents among people with learning disabilities, negative attitudes of professionals towards people and communication difficulties (Kiani et al 2014). Of course, cancer does not present differently in people with learning disabilities. Health professionals can be distracted from the task at hand by diagnostic overshadowing which I return to later in this chapter.

People with learning disabilities are more commonly affected by gastroesophageal reflux disease, which includes constipation, gastritis and bowel obstruction-related deaths, than the wider population (Haveman et al 2010). This is likely due to a combination of a lack of exercise and healthy diet (which I return to in Chapter 5) and long-term medication use, although it is also attributed to having an IQ less than 35 (Haveman et al 2010). It is peculiar that a non-scientific, and as we saw in Chapter 1, nonsensical measurement can be presented as a cause of ill-health. It is also possible to identify circulating narratives of 'strange' and 'otherworldly' in these 'scientific' publications, which work as a mechanism to allow health professionals to continue to treat patients with learning disabilities differently and pay little attention to poor outcomes or death.

Returning to the evidence trail, a meta-analysis of hospital care in England and Australia identified delayed prescription of epilepsy medication, lack of support to eat (including being given the right utensils to eat), to go to toilet or move from the bed and 'endemic' discriminatory attitudes towards people with learning disabilities (Bradbury-Jones et al 2013).

Krahn et al (2006) developed a cascade model with the prevalence of observable health conditions in people with learning disabilities such as early onset dementia and epilepsy at the top. Subsequent layers feature absences or disparities in attention to care needs; in preventative care and health promotion practices; and in equitable access to healthcare. This model was later extended using a review of international literature around the health disparities people with learning disabilities experience published between 2002 and 2011 (Krahn and Fox 2014). An optimistic picture is presented going forward as the authors suggest improvements in surveillance and data generation will provide opportunities to maximize the impact of interventions. This optimism appears thin a decade on with little evidence these opportunities are taken up and used.

Communication error is identified as a major factor (70%) in adverse events involving people with learning disabilities, although this measure is criticised as simplistic and in need of more precise unpacking (Guttman et al 2021). There is support for this criticism in the following extract by US academic Davy (2019 p109) writing about the key role families play in the healthcare of relatives with learning disabilities, in this case, the hospitalisation of her sister. The lack of narrative humility is all too apparent:

> Over a period of a few days, my family and I had learnt to translate the tiny, hidden signs of Millie's pain: a furrow between her eyebrows or her molars grinding together almost imperceptibly. Removed from the rhythm and music of her daily life, she was unable to make her voice heard. The doctors and nurses were too unfamiliar with her or too busy to learn to listen. At that moment, by her bedside, I was the only one with the depth of knowledge and understanding of her to represent her pain to others.

We find, repeatedly, it is family members or people with learning disabilities who engage in narrative humility, who listen, pay attention, love and care for and about family members. They often take this work further by acting on their knowledge and understanding and advocating for their family members and wider (Runswick-Cole et al. 2024, Ryan and Runswick-Cole 2009).

I finish this brief literature review with a report by the Nuffield Trust (2024) which offers a contemporary summary of the health experiences of people with learning disabilities in England. This report found people were more likely to be obese, less likely to be involved in screening programmes for breast and cervical cancer, more likely to receive a cancer diagnosis later than the wider population and to have poorer access to mental health services. Furthermore, only 26% of the (known about) population of people with learning disabilities are estimated to be on the learning disability register in general practitioner (GP) surgeries which hinders the uptake of annual health checks.

The landscape of abhorrence has a particularly grim shade when it comes to healthcare practices and people with learning disabilities. The evidence base reads as having a veneer of 'do better' while practice remains largely untroubled and unchanged. Indeed, while writing this book, the Labour government have withdrawn their commitment to increasing the number of people with learning disabilities having an annual health check to 75%. As Krahn and Fox (2014) argued a decade ago, poor health outcomes among people with learning disabilities should be considered intolerable rather than a given. We remain all too practiced in tolerating them.

Annual health checks

So let us turn to consider the intervention that is recommended internationally as a health policy component (Robertson et al 2014) and implemented in several countries, including Australia, the Netherlands and the United Kingdom. An annual health check with GPs, or in some cases, primary care staff, provides a specific and targeted opportunity to review the health and wellbeing of people with learning disabilities, and potentially identify developing health conditions or needs. In Australia, the Comprehensive Health Assessment Program (CHAP) was introduced after the government set up a Medicare rebate for annual health checks in 2007. It is a 29-page form that should be completed by the patient, their support worker or family member and the GP. In England, health checks were introduced in primary care in 2008 based on a recommendation by the Disability Rights Commission (2006), although they were used previously. An earlier study, for example, introduced health checks by a GP and consultant psychiatrist in one GP surgery in England and found the intervention was useful in picking up unmet health needs (Cassidy et al 2002).

Since the incentivised (which is a key component) roll out of annual health checks in England, people with learning disabilities aged 14 and over are supposed to be included in a GP register which flags the need for annual checks. National Institute for Clinical Excellence (NICE) guidelines suggest these checks should include a review of the person's physical and mental health, medication use, vaccinations, secondary care coordination arrangements, transition arrangements if appropriate, a review of communication needs, family carer needs and supporting people to look after their health (NICE Quality Standards 2015).

Health checks can be effective in identifying a range of issues from serious and life-threatening conditions to more minor conditions (Robertson et al 2014). They can reduce the high risk of emergency hospitalisation (Carey et al 2017) and are not costly in practice (Gordon et al 2012). As is often the case, improvements in healthcare services may not require complicated, costly or unreasonable efforts. Other evidence suggests health checks have improved access to healthcare. For example, an analysis of Scottish healthcare records across two time periods in the last two decades shows some reduction in the health inequality gap in the management of long-term conditions for people with learning disabilities, although overall management remained poorer than for the wider population (Hughes-McCormack et al 2022). The authors suggest the programme of health checks and learning disability health service support may have contributed to this improvement.

A meta-ethnographic review of experiences of health checks found people very much wanted to be actively involved in their healthcare, although there was confusion around the purpose of health checks and what they may signify (Gregson et al 2022). This review, which included papers from the United States, United Kingdom, Netherlands, Canada, Wales and Scotland, flagged up the importance of trust, organisational access, communication and adjustments, as well as discriminatory staff attitudes. I feel I should have introduced a game of recommendation bingo for the reader as the same issues are identified and recommendations repeatedly presented as the solution. More refreshingly, Gregson et al (2022) identified a shift in how people with learning disabilities were represented in the articles from 2009 when they started to be described as more active and capable in relation to their healthcare, suggesting an improvement in attitudes. Of course, a broad change that is needed is the involvement of people with learning disabilities in their lives, their healthcare, their relationships, housing, work and research. Without this involvement, people will continue to be misunderstood and treated as not fully human, and the cycle of impoverishment will continue.

Uptake of health checks remains low internationally despite it being a simple and clear intervention with considerable potential impact. The barriers to uptake offer further evidence of disregard and ignorance on the part of healthcare professionals; a lack of awareness about health assessments and a lack of training in conducting the assessment. Practitioners identified a lack of skills, knowledge and confidence in this area. Other excuses include time constraints, practitioner burnout and not being able to find patients with learning disabilities among the electronic systems (Caltabiano et al 2024). Indeed, one study reported that GPs did not know the code to add patients with learning disabilities to the GP register (Bakker-van Gijssel et al 2017).

Self-identifying a lack of skills, knowledge or confidence in providing healthcare to a group of patients should generate efforts to rectify this gap, to learn these skills and develop confidence. Not knowing a key code to flag certain patients on electronic records is a failing in practice that should not be tolerated. We saw earlier how nearly 75% of people with learning disabilities are not on the GP register in England. While some GPs recognise the importance of health checks and are eager to provide preventative healthcare (Caltabiano et al 2024), the wider and again lacklustre attention to detail extends to recording information relating to the health check which can be varied with little attention paid to mental health or medication reviews (Carey et al 2017).

Recommendations around health checks co-produced with people with learning disabilities offer fresh perspectives and include changing the term 'annual health check' to yearly health check to make it clear people with learning disabilities can see their GP outside of this check (Wigham et al 2022). It is not always clear if people have had a health check. For example, P8, in one study, described how:

> I'm not quite sure [if I've had an annual healthcheck], but I need to see a doctor.
> *(Cooper-Moss et al 2024 np)*

As health inequalities are a human rights and social justice issue, it is a clear contravention of these that an incentivised, mandated intervention with national guidelines about content and process remains so poorly implemented.

Diagnostic overshadowing

The next area I focus on in this chapter is another feature of (failing) healthcare for people with learning disabilities: diagnostic overshadowing. I also consider intersectionality here because there is overlap between the two concepts. We saw in Chapter 1 how even social theorists of marginalised groups ignore or overlook people with learning disabilities, a baffling omission given the contribution this area could make to the robustness of theoretical approaches. Goodey (2017 p26) puzzles over this absence:

> Is it just accidental forgetting, or is it because people with learning difficulties (let's say in this case profound or severe ones) do not even qualify as an *out*group, let alone an ingroup? In other words, the people thus labelled do not in the last resort qualify as human.

Research about, sometimes with, people with learning disabilities can ignore or overlook intersectionality, an omission which could be interpreted as a form of research overshadowing or poor academic practice. This leaves the evidence base around the experiences and lives of people with learning disabilities further compromised, adding layers of disrespect to already disrespected lives, as well as the potential for harm. We know people with learning disabilities from ethnic minority backgrounds experience additional obstacles accessing healthcare, including a lack of cultural and religious sensitivity and communication barriers (Cooper-Moss et al 2024, NHS Race and Health Observatory 2023).

One study in Norway highlighted how immigrant families with a child with learning disabilities can experience greater challenges in terms of accessing information, social isolation and post-migration challenges. Cultural ignorance, discrimination and limited social networks are apparent (Nyikach and Hansen 2024). One participant, Zalman, described how:

> Another important thing I want to say is this: I am not like an ordinary ethnic Norwegian who has a disabled child. I am a foreigner with painful experiences of wars and torture. I have experienced strange things that I cannot tell you. Every single one of them was traumatic. These things have made me suspicious of authorities. I can say that my daughter is also a victim of the terrible situations I went through. I worry about her future.
>
> *(Nyikach and Hansen 2024 p194)*

Immigrant families experience a lack of accessible information, understanding, cultural barriers that risk receiving no, or the wrong, support or treatment and professionals are ill equipped to negotiate this. In the United Kingdom, little is known about the experiences of people with learning disabilities from ethnic minorities (Robertson et al 2019). A qualitative synthesis of literature published since 1990 found families with a relative with learning disabilities from ethnic minority backgrounds experience conflicts of control in accessing healthcare around culture and choice, as well as racism, although the latter is rarely discussed in terms of what this means for people with learning disabilities (Roberts et al 2024). The synthesis also found an absence of consideration of other sociopolitical and systematic factors such as socioeconomic status.

The intersection of gender, learning disabilities and mental health has not been the focus of much attention although recent research suggests women with learning disabilities are further disadvantaged when accessing mental health services (Whittle et al 2024). A study of linked datasets in New South Wales found no difference between women and men in relation to socio-economic class suggesting gender is less prominent in relation to learning disability. The findings reflected the gendered nature of the diagnosis of mental ill health in the wider population with women with learning disabilities being more likely to be diagnosed with depression, anxiety and mood disorders. Women with learning disabilities were also more likely to experience diagnostic instability suggesting they have a more complicated journey to receiving a reliable diagnosis and, subsequently, appropriate treatment. Wider research about disabled women found sociocultural, financial and structural facts which impacts their access to healthcare (Matin et al 2021).

Diagnostic overshadowing refers to the attribution of signs and symptoms of mental or physical illness to the label of learning disabilities (Ali et al 2013, Mason and Scior 2004), and was initially highlighted in the early 1980s (Reiss et al 1982). While the identification of this failing could have been used as a lever for improved practice, the term has become an abstraction used to normalise the abnormal and explain away poor practice. A clinical example of the use of the term is provided by Javaid et al (2019 p8):

> Diagnostic overshadowing is increasingly recognised as contributing to health inequalities experienced by the learning disability population. This case is that of a 54-year-old male with mild-to-moderate learning disability who displayed abnormally aggressive behaviours and self-neglect. He had multiple transfers between the psychiatric and medical units during an inpatient episode, partly due to his physical health symptoms being misattributed to learning disability and challenging behaviour.

Diagnostic overshadowing is an example of ignorance underpinned by assumptions that should play no role in healthcare. It is an outcome of a lack of critical engagement, knowledge, thought and sense. Health professionals often do not know or refuse to know what they should know, fill these knowledge gaps with assumptions and act on these assumptions.

The acknowledgement of the term in clinical (and wider) practice is a further example of epistemic injustice, of not listening to people. The failure to listen to people, their family members or support workers sits alongside ignorance about the experiences of being a person with learning disabilities, or a family carer of a person with learning disabilities. That these experiences remain largely absent from our collective understanding is a form of structural discrimination. Unsurprisingly, the constant call for more awareness among practitioners is repeated in this area (Wigham et al 2022).

Over-medication of psychotropic medicines and a low rate of medicine reviews are an associated strand of diagnostic overshadowing. These have been reported in several countries, including the United Kingdom (Cavanagh et al 2024), Netherlands (de Kuijper et al 2010) and Spain (Folch et al 2019). Prescribing medication in the absence of a formal psychiatric diagnosis contravenes acceptable medical practice in England and yet is common for people with learning disabilities, where an estimated 30,000–35,000 people with learning disabilities are prescribed medication by their GP without clinical justification (Glover et al 2015). Patients and family carers are poorly informed about this prescription and the associated side-effects (Cavanagh et al 2024). This is a further example of the contradiction, embedded absurdity and systemic failings in the healthcare of people with learning disabilities; being prescribed medication without a formal mental ill-health diagnosis and not receiving an annual health check, including a medication review, because people are not flagged on the GP register. It suggests wilful participation in a highly selective and spurious use of 'medical expertise' on the part of health professionals. At some point in the development of the systemic operation of healthcare systems, in this instance, the NHS, it became acceptable for people with learning disabilities to be subjected to over-medication of psychotropic medicines with few or no questions asked, even post-death as I return to later in this chapter.

People with learning disabilities are ignored, 'done to' and dismissed in an array of spaces and settings, including healthcare. This silencing, this testimonial epistemic injustice, has various implications. The imprecise record or account of symptoms can lead to serious illness remaining untreated and premature death. There can be a cumulative impact on confidence and speaking up, or even courage which leaves people subject to neglect and abuse (Dohmen 2016). Fricker (2007 p130) uses the term 'pre-emptive testimonial injustice' to describe instances where people do not share information because they are silenced by others who do not seek their knowledge. People are epistemologically objectified as pre-emptive testimonial injustice is woven into the fabric of their lives through micro-aggressions which include being overlooked, disrespected and discounted from a young age. Indeed, if people try to engage, to share their feelings or experiences, the outcome can be a label of 'challenging behaviour', as we saw above, reinforcing disciplinary power (Mikulak et al 2024, Sirotkin 2024).

It is possible to attend to the needs and health of people, including those with profound learning disabilities as Dohmen (2016) outlines, offering uncomplicated suggestions; paying attention to and taking seriously expressions of pleasure, pain, preferences and dislikes, listening to what those people close to the person say and fostering the development of epistemic capabilities as much as possible. While there is acknowledgement of inequalities around operationalising the latter point as it is likely that people with social and economic capital are better placed to do this, these suggestions support the concept of narrative humility and again, speak to the simplicity around what needs to change. The self-identified lack of knowledge, confidence and skills practitioners report could be ameliorated by asking the person, their support worker or family carer how they can best help. Just two examples from the 'pockets of brilliance' tweets demonstrate this simplicity (Ryan 2020 p37):

> Recovery ward making sure Ear Defenders were put on straight after op, machines silenced and lights down low, curtains shut and that I was there before 20 yo woke then put in a side ward. (Superstes – @freedom4lou)

> Never forget nurse who arranged for the big prince to have his own room for cardiology appts. He arrived to a drs room with his name on the door, access to a computer & WiFi. Drs came to his room not theirs! Anxiety plummeted!! (Marianne SB – @mariannesb37)

Dying too soon

Enduring discrepancies between the mortality rates of people with learning disabilities and their non-disabled peers offer further evidence of health and social care failings, and systemic discriminatory practices. While some people with learning disabilities may have an increased risk of developing certain health conditions as discussed earlier, being diagnosed with learning disabilities as a baby or young child should not dictate a shortened lifetime.

In England, the '*Stop People Dying Too Young*' group of self-advocates has campaigned for changes to healthcare access for people with learning disabilities to prevent premature deaths. One member, Gavin said:

> Our lives have as much value as everyone else's. We are all unique and individual. We are not a diagnosis or a label. People should see the person, not the disability or what race I am.

Another UK-based self-advocacy group, My Life My Choice, runs a campaign called 'We Can't Wait' demanding people with learning disabilities are moved up higher on hospital waiting lists to reduce the number of people dying early. As the campaign Champion, Kumudu Perera says, "it's not about jumping queues, it's about saving lives".

This activism is necessary as wider health inequalities and associated premature deaths in England have remained the same or worsened despite considerable research and policy attention (Smith et al 2016, Tyrer and McGrother 2009). The latest LEDER report shows that the average age of death for people with learning disabilities in England is 62.9 (White et al 2023), in contrast to 82.8 years for women and 78.8 years for non-disabled men (ONS 2021). People with learning disabilities from ethnic minority backgrounds have a life expectancy of half of that of white people with learning disabilities, with an average age of death at 34 years (O'Dowd 2023). People continue to die from unfathomable and preventative health conditions such as constipation, choking and drowning (Laugharne et al 2024, Ryan 2017).

Evidence about premature and preventable deaths is compelling, contradictory and sometimes confusing. This is in part due to incomplete data or what I go on to describe in a later section, 'dodgy data' based on assumption-led research and the tweaking of regulatory and mandatory death-reporting processes to overlook the deaths of people with learning disabilities.

So what does some of the research tell us? An international systematic review found people with profound learning disabilities had poorer mortality rates compared to the general population, and women with learning disabilities experience greater inequalities than men with learning disabilities with the main causes of death being respiratory and circulatory diseases (O'Leary et al 2018). The 27 papers included in the review were based on research conducted in the Global North. While people with learning disabilities in the United States have similar health risks such as cancer and heart disease to non-disabled people, pneumonia, influenza and choking are common causes of death (Landes et al 2020). A quantitative study of people with learning disabilities who died in Ireland between 2001 and 2016 found the mean age of death rose from 47.1 years in 2001 to 53.1 years by 2016, women again had a higher mean age of death than men and while the age at death increased, the inequality gap remained the same (Doyle et al 2021). The odds of people dying who live in congregate (group) settings were four times higher than those living with family members, suggesting less care and attention is paid to people living in these often-considerably costly and supposedly regulated services. The authors conclude there is no evidence these discrepancies are closing and despite many avoidable deaths, preventative actions do not seem to have been taken. In Scotland, children and young people with learning disabilities are more likely to die of all-cause, avoidable, treatable and preventable causes than their non-disabled peers (Hughes-McCormack et al 2022).

The recommendations of a Swedish population-based cohort study include health advocacy programmes to support people's comprehension and communication, improved take-up of screening programmes and the promotion of active participation in health encounters (Hirvikoski et al 2021). And so it continues – more recommendations about identifying people with learning disabilities in national health registers, more health checks and training for health professionals. It is important to note again the consistent focus among these recommendations on changing the person with learning disabilities rather than addressing wider structural oppression.

In England, a clear path can be traced from report to inquiry to report since the publication of *Healthcare for All* (Michael 2008). This report offered ten, some again well-rehearsed, recommendations which included amending the Core Standards for Better Health to reflect requirement to make 'reasonable adjustments' to services, partnership working with people with learning disabilities and families to plan care, staff training, stronger regulatory practices and the establishment of a National Confidential Inquiry.

The Confidential Inquiry into the deaths of People with Learning Disabilities commissioned after this report published its findings in 2013. The 18 recommendations, some of which overlapped with the *Healthcare for All* recommendations, included setting up a National Mortality Review Board to scrutinise unexpected deaths. A National Confidential Enquiry into Maternal Deaths established in England and Wales in 1952, led to a significant fall in maternal mortality and versions of such inquiries exist in various countries, including Japan, the USA, Russia and the Netherlands (Drife et al 2023). The government, however, rebutted the recommendation saying it was too costly, thereby adding another strand of cost-saving evidence for the conditions of social murder.

These developments and non-developments underline the little genuine interest in or commitment to improving the healthcare and treatment of people with learning disabilities. When we see broader concern, it is more often a response to a particular scandal such as Winterbourne View in England (Flynn and Citarella 2013), the Huronia Regional Centre in Canada (Rossiter and Clarkson 2013) or the Esidemenis scandal in South Africa (Capri et al 2018). These scandals typically involve large numbers of people with learning disabilities or, in the case of Winterbourne View, a privately run assessment and treatment unit in the West of England, documentary film footage of cruelty and abuse by staff towards residents.

A minimum of 140 people with learning disabilities or people with mental ill health died after funding for the Esidemenis Life institution was cut by the Gauteng Department of Health in 2015. This led to the discharge and dispersal of people with high support needs to inappropriate support settings, despite efforts made by family members and organisations to prevent this happening (Ferlito and Dhai 2018). Capri et al (2018 p153) describe how, while these deaths are abominable, the mark of a 'silent catastrophe' implies the abuse of people matters less than dying through neglect; dead or alive is the only meaningful statistic which means the lives people lead are irrelevant.

I suggest that being neglected to death, while noteworthy on a larger scale or through filmed evidence, has a temporally limited impact which puts it on a continuum with abuse rather than eclipsing it. Neither matter or count in the longer term. These scandals force performative action on the part of government or other institutions which is downgraded over time as the scandal is quietly unmade, facilitated by the collective of politicians, policy makers, health and social care providers and professionals, researchers and national charities, alongside an almost countless number of moral bystanders.

A clear example of this is the unmaking of the momentary scandal around Connor's death (Ryan 2017). An independent review was commissioned by NHS England into the deaths of people with learning disabilities, older people and people with mental ill health between 2011 and 2015 in the NHS hospital where

Connor died. This was the outcome of a grassroots campaign for accountability in relation to his death called #JusticeForLB (Connor was affectionately known as Laughing Boy). Mazars, a global consultancy, conducted the review which produced grotesque evidence of the discounting of unexpected deaths and the seamless ability to ignore standard investigatory protocols and procedures. For example, less than 1% of the unexpected deaths of people with learning disabilities were investigated. The health of people with learning disabilities was viewed as inherently compromised by hospital staff who did not follow clear and well-documented procedures around investigating unexpected deaths. Publication of the report was delayed for several months in 2015. The NHS Trust strongly challenged the findings, and NHS England subsequently commissioned a review into the review.

The second review was conducted by a Bristol University team who asked for further details of the workings out that underpinned the analysis to be included in the report. The Bristol team concluded the findings were robust. NHS England continued to delay publication of the report until a copy was leaked to the BBC and published in December 2015. Then Health Secretary Jeremy Hunt was called to the House of Commons to face cross-party condemnation of the report's findings and promised to set up a new *Learning from Deaths* programme to address the issues raised by the review across the 215 NHS Trusts in England. Within months, the focus on people with learning disabilities and/or mental ill health disappeared and the programme became a wider intervention in relation to the reporting of hospital deaths (Ryan 2017).

The Mazars report revealed how some lives and deaths do not count and what are considered to be clear and robust statutory investigatory processes can be systematically ignored. Indeed, the NHS hospital reported Connor died of natural causes in their board minutes less than three weeks after his death (Ryan 2017). The process of undertaking the Mazars review further revealed mechanisms of power and epistemic injustices within public sector bodies such as NHS organisations. The investigation uncovered extraordinary evidence which led to belligerent ignorance and the associated explicit forms of resistance by the NHS hospital and national NHS body that commissioned the review. And yet, the scandal was unmade in the months that followed leaving a further injustice; that the wider population can benefit from interventions generated from the mistreatment of people with learning disabilities without changes to the lives of people with learning disabilities.

Death reporting and investigatory processes

People with learning disabilities continue to experience avoidable deaths and the failings of harm-related investigatory processes in this area that extend to death reporting and investigatory processes. Deaths can be badged as 'natural causes' leading to no further investigation with acknowledged apathy around not bothering to look too closely into what happened (Julian 2020).

In several countries, including the United Kingdom and the United States, death certificates are divided into two parts. Part 1 asks for the specific cause of death to be recorded, and Part 2, for detail of any other conditions that contribute to the death but are not part of the sequence of events leading to death. Learning disability is not a cause of death and yet continues to be represented as such on death certificates. Landes et al (2020), for example, found almost half of the death certificates of people with learning disabilities in the United States had learning disability reported as their underlying cause of death, while in Finland learning disability was mentioned in 38.9% of death certificates (Patja et al 2001). There were also instances of underreporting when the learning disability directly or indirectly contributed to the death (Landes et al 2020). Being in a position to certify deaths underlines the power and privilege of the medical profession, and integrity, truthfulness and responsibility is essential. The investigation into the Life Esidemeni scandal found 85% of death certificates stated natural causes which meant medical officers either ignored or did not notice signs of neglect (Dhai 2018).

A further issue is that death certification (outside of cause of death sections) does not always include mention of learning disability which has implications for the scrutiny of the deaths of people with learning disabilities (Carey et al 2017). This is the same for Prevention of Future Death reports issued by coroners which I return to below. Imprecise reporting overlooks deaths from preventable causes, removing opportunities for learning and further undermining the reliability of mortality trends. This could also be interpreted as a type of diagnostic death overshadowing as the constant surveillance people with learning disabilities experience across their lives, abruptly stops when they die.

At Connor's inquest, there was shock and incredulity in the second week of the hearing when it was disclosed by the NHS hospital that another patient with learning disabilities, Henry, died in the same bath as Connor some years earlier (Ryan 2017). That his death was disclosed so late in an investigatory process that had taken over two years was extraordinary. What visibly shocked the coroner was that Henry's death was not investigated and there was no inquest. His death was certified as natural causes by a hospital consultant (who was present on the day Connor died), and no further investigation took place. Henry was 56 years old.

Given how endemic this misreporting and covering up is, we should ask why and how ignorance is apparent in these situations, and what this ignorance is doing. It could imply lurking concerns that the person did not receive appropriate treatment hence the lack of scrutiny. We could draw on Goodey's interpretation of people not qualifying as human in which case there is no need for an investigation into how the non-person died, the death investigatory processes do not apply. Death investigations further have resource implications which can be avoided if the rules do not apply. The same logic that leads to the mistreatment and abuse of people applies after they die.

This misrepresentation or cover up does many things. It leads to the generation of what I call dodgy data which stops patterns and trends of deaths from being identified. It creates falsehoods and sustains assumptions that people with learning disabilities die earlier than people without learning disabilities which, in turn, creates a loop of expecting and accepting premature deaths. Connor's death and the subsequent Mazar's review disrupted this loop albeit momentarily. The LEDER annual death review process continues to report scandalous findings which are barely reported in the wider media. The public memory is all too lax to join any dots in this area.

Knowledge transfer consultant and journalist, Dr George Julian, has live-tweeted UK-based inquests of people with learning disabilities and/or autism since Connor's inquest in October 2015. Summaries are published at www.georgejulian.co.uk/blog/. This decade of documentary journalism offers further evidence about how people with learning disabilities do not matter. Expert witnesses can offer repeated examples of discounting or denying failures in what is often basic healthcare and treatment, providing 'evidence' that repeatedly points to the assumption that people with learning disabilities will die earlier (of natural causes), that there is something inherently flawed about them so when they do, investigations can be light or no touch. There are sometimes identifiable hints of incredulity or indignation in the reporting of the responses of these experts to questioning by the coroner or, more often, family counsel, of their expertise being challenged.

In a study of how bereaved families experience the English coronial process when the relative was autistic, had learning disabilities and/or mental ill health, we found epistemic courage and resistance was needed on the part of family members. Expert witnesses often exercised their epistemic privilege regardless of how knowledgeable they were (Ryan et al 2024b). The knowledge of the coroner, imbued by seniority and official authority, could be central to this ignorance. Julian's longitudinal work, however, demonstrates how some coroners who lead repeated inquests into the deaths of people with learning disabilities and/or autistic people begin to develop a sharper understanding and awareness. In effect, they begin to demonstrate narrative humility through careful listening and paying care and attention to family members, drawing on strategies to reduce testimonial injustices. These enlightened coroners become more resistant to accepting the absurd as explanations for the paucity of effective healthcare and begin to challenge problematic actions by health or social care professionals.

Findings of serious failings in the English coronial system can lead to the coroner issuing a Prevention of Future Deaths report which are publicly logged online at www.judiciary.uk/?s=&pfd_report_type=&post_type=pfd&order=relevance.

The organisation involved, which may be an NHS hospital, local authority, care provider, prison service or police force, must respond to this report within a particular timeframe. A review of these reports, however, suggests little apparent learning and, subsequently, repeated deaths from the same causes. Leary et al (2021) further found layers of shoddiness in, for example, the cut and pasting of text across responses. Another mandatory process which is clearly not fit for practice and yet remains unchallenged.

These reports which are searchable on the Courts and Tribunals Judiciary website offer incontrovertible evidence of how people are failed in life and subsequently in death. For example, one young woman, Juliet Saunders, was 25 when she died from neglect after attending the Accident and Emergency department at Barking and Havering NHS University hospital in 2021. The coroner's report details the lack of any support for people with learning disabilities at the weekend when learning disability nurses are not on duty, poor medical record keeping and supervision of junior doctors, abnormal scan findings were overlooked due to diagnostic overshadowing, a lack of clinical curiosity led to bowel obstruction remaining undiagnosed, there was no safety netting advice on discharge and an investigation into Juliet's death was ineffective (Judiciary UK 2021). The routine list of failings that appear on PFD reports (bearing in mind so few of the preventable deaths of people with learning disabilities will make it into the coronial process) become almost embarrassing evidence for social murder. I say embarrassing because it is inconceivable that a list of such failures attributed to the death of a non-marginalised person would not attract serious attention and inquiry.

The evidence around the premature and preventable deaths of people with learning disabilities is clear with the caveat again that this evidence is largely based in higher income countries and much remains uninvestigated and reported. People with learning disabilities do not receive the protection their fellow citizens are entitled to and the mortality gap between people with learning disabilities and the mainstream population remains consistent. As Medina (2018) argues, epistemologies of ignorance lead to profound forms of epistemic injustice. Too many are invested in misunderstanding or ignoring the obvious; that social murder is happening in full view.

Research exclusion and other problematic practices

In the final section in this chapter, I want to explore the contributions academics, funders, ethics committees and journal editors make to the uneven evidence base in this area and, thereby, help to sustain oppressive practices. As McDonnell and Phelan (2022 p5) argue,

> A concern is that while researchers have challenged the association of intellectual disability with unfitness, they have rarely challenged—and may have inadvertently reified—normative assumptions of embodiment and citizenship, which give rise to attributions of incapacity.

To begin with, research focus and questions can firmly position people with learning disabilities as not fully human. Systematic reviews have been published of the effects of exercise on the fitness levels of people with learning disabilities (Bouzas et al 2019), and secondary health conditions, health promotion and employment in relation to people with learning disabilities (Iwanaga et al 2021). The latter article is a systematic review of systematic reviews. These studies found: exercise benefits people with learning disabilities; people are more at risk of secondary health conditions; health promotion can make a difference; and people have a better quality of life if they are employed. The idea that exercise, health promotion and employment may not be beneficial for people with learning disabilities suggests that people are seen as other than human.

I'm reminded of a story Goodey (2017 p11) recounts about parents asking if their child with learning disabilities could attend a mainstream primary school near where they lived. The headteacher says no, the child would disrupt the other children because they would not be able to sit quietly in assembly. When challenged by the parents that many children do not sit quietly in assembly, the headteacher shifts to present other excuses. Goodey uses this example of absurdity, drawing on Tajfel (1981), to demonstrate how stereotypical categorisations become delusional and impose a forced choice of definitional criteria on professionals. I suggest this includes researchers. In a lighter moment, in writing *Love, Learning Disabilities and Brilliance*, and tweeting about this story, one parent carer replied saying she had a similar experience with a headteacher;

> Sounds identical to the conversation we had … school where I had been a member of staff before it split into infant and junior so new infant head. We got an answer eventually – it's epilepsy – 'tuts' – PE – wall bars…
>
> *(Ryan 2020 p31)*

It does not take much work to find evidence of the silencing of people with learning disabilities in the underlining assumptions and pejorative judgements implicitly and explicitly made by researchers and research teams, and accepted by various academic stakeholders, including funding bodies, ethics committees and journal editorial boards. Just one example, in a study that involved people with learning disabilities as participants, demonstrates the pejorative tone that can be used:

> They [people with learning disabilities] complained about communication problems and difficulties understanding medical jargon. However, they did not seem to relate their health problems to their lifestyles, and there was an absence of any kind of responsibility for their own health.
>
> *(Tilly 2013, p228)*

Equity in access to appropriate and timely healthcare will not be possible while people with learning disabilities continue to be systematically excluded from research involvement (Shepherd 2020, Shepherd et al 2022). This speaks to hermeneutical injustice and the lack of knowledge and understanding in collective resources. Research, including clinical trial participation, should represent the groups likely to use the findings, medical product or intervention under investigation. We know key causes of death in people with learning disabilities in

England relate to respiratory and circulatory disorders and yet people are denied the right to participate in research in these (and wider) areas.

A review of 26,293 studies in England recorded in the government-funded National Institute for Health Research (now Health and Care Research) portfolio to determine the inclusion of people with learning disabilities in this funded research body found 60.3% of studies listed 'learning disability' as an exclusion criterion (Spaul et al 2020) and these findings are likely to be underestimates. No studies researching pneumonia or sepsis included people with learning disabilities. The authors conclude a review of ethical barriers is needed with more scrutiny by research-funding organisations of the justifications provided for these exclusions. UK funding councils are presented as rigorous and unbiased and yet blanket exclusions in nearly 16,000 research projects were not challenged by funding committees. The exclusion criteria were approved by ethics committees and were not discussed as potential research limitations in research publications, widening the ring of ignorance to peer reviewers and journal editors. Indeed, ethics committees can demonstrate biomedical understandings of disability and infantilise people with learning disabilities with the apparent intention of protection (Jones 2021, Santinele Martino and Schormans 2018).

Learning disability is an exclusion criterion *and* a cause of death: a label that does some heavy lifting. So, where does our theorising take us here? Is this an example of hermeneutical epistemic injustice, of overwhelming systematic discrimination against people who are again, to re-quote Goodey (2017), so far outside the outgroup, they do not qualify as human? It is certainly a form of contributory injustice as people are denied the opportunity to take part in research without any apparent reflection. It also speaks to ignorance on the part of the research community who accept the dressing up of the social and political construction of learning disability as a neutral and natural fact that applies to certain people (Altermark 2017). We saw in Chapter 1 how academics can accept people with learning disabilities are different and see that difference as somehow resting in their condition (Carey 2009). The often-quoted statement "if you have met one autistic person, you have met one autistic person" by Dr Stephen Shore (Flannery and Wisner-Carlson 2020) applies to people with learning disabilities and yet the research community parcels people up into a homogenous package, ties a bow around it and deposits it as being explicitly outside of research thought, consideration and practice.

These exclusions have been explained, in part, as an outcome of the different legal frameworks underpinning research governance and practice which vary within and between countries (Shepherd 2020). In the United Kingdom, there is, further, a lack of understanding and expertise around these frameworks and interpretations of the Mental Capacity Act (Shepherd 2020). While the Council for International Organizations of Medical Sciences has updated international ethics guidance, marking a shift to having to *justify* exclusion, this is not yet reflected in legal frameworks, and it remains difficult to gain ethical approval to include people who lack capacity (Shepherd 2020).

We overcame this challenge in *Growing Older,* after initial resistance from the university ethics team, by arguing people with learning disabilities have the right to take part in research (Michael 2021, Shepherd 2020), particularly in research about them or about issues that directly affect them. Like the enlightened coroners described above, it seems that one way forward is for these individual actions on a case-by-case basis to chip away at assumptions. Indeed, there is a developing body of thoughtful and critical reflections around negotiating ethics and ethics committees in this field with the underlying aim of supporting other researchers to improve their practice (see, for example, Thomas 2024 and Jones 2021).

The consequences of this exclusion are again manifold. People have the right to participate in and benefit from evidence-based care. Excluding certain groups from research can lead to distorted findings which can unjustly disadvantage those groups (Michael 2021). This is another form of epistemic exclusion where people are not only excluded from research participation, the process of generating knowledge, but are denied the opportunity to challenge decisions around healthcare allocation because they will likely be unaware that they are adversely affected by decisions in this area (Michael 2021). Healthcare committees and professionals may work towards evidence-based guidance assuming the underlying evidence is accurate and valid and if the evidence, for example, underpinning rationing decisions is flawed, this can feed into enduring inequalities. It also isolates people with learning disabilities who are denied the opportunity to contribute to research, and as a consequence, wider society.

Suggestions to address this imbalance include a mechanism to specifically involve people which is something funding councils are addressing albeit for varying reasons (see, for example, Russell et al 2019), more forensic examination of disinvestment decisions and an independent process to represent marginalised groups.

At the beginning of this chapter, I discussed Popay's (2010) call to arms among public health colleagues and the criticality of the nursing profession demonstrating moral courage (McGibbon and Lukeman 2019). I suspect the epistemic ignorance demonstrated by some researchers is underpinned by not knowing or understanding much, or anything, about learning disability, as well as working within siloes of narrow interests. There may be assumptions that people with learning disabilities are unable to participate in research or have nothing of value to contribute, that it is too hard within funded research timetables to work out ways of engaging with people, of adjusting research designs to accommodate participation. Researchers may be reluctant to take on what can be intimidating ethics committees. Jones (2021), for example, reports having to respond to 18 email-based enquiries in the process of gaining ethics approval for her doctoral research. This is a social justice issue, however, and the academic community should do better and do more to redress this. As Ginn (2022 p932) argues, we have a responsibility about who we hold accountable for change, and a crucial role to play in shaping policies, institutions and practice.

A further issue in relation to research practice is the optimism researchers within the field of learning disability express in relation to their recommendations (which is something I have done). We tend to be optimistic about changes in the future with little evidence of changes from the past. Thomson et al (2021), for example, conducted a systematic review into the impact of intentional sports programmes on community participation and found these programmes did not translate into more community participation in the wider community. The authors conclude "significant research" is required to work out how it could. Bradbury-Jones et al (2013 p1507) conclude there must be "a genuine desire to improve the health, safety and welfare of adults with learning disabilities". These statements can be traced back across decades and read as whimsical when placed within the context of the enduring inequalities people face. Research recommendations tend to focus on changing the lives of people with learning disabilities rather than addressing the restrictions people face (Ginn 2022). In relation to her work on historic violence, Mohamed (2024 p5) describes how researchers can presume that readers do not know about these violences and once we present the evidence to the world, people will think differently and act,

> In so doing, we create epistemic innocence when what we may be confronted by are unethical epistemes and unethical readers who are invested in misunderstanding and ignoring the obvious.

Repeatedly documented failings in basic health and social care should generate a more critical engagement, as evidence by Miner et al (2024 p1),

> As nursing and midwifery professionals, have we met the enemy and are we willing to acknowledge that as educators, clinicians, scholars, and system leaders we represent major barriers to improving health equity for persons with intellectual and developmental disabilities? Are we willing to admit that, despite the call for action to 'Close the gap' from the Office of the Surgeon General US [...] more than two decades ago and repeated calls since then [...], we fail to address PWIDD's [people with intellectual and developmental disability] healthcare needs?

We can conduct what can be distorted scholarship (Medina 2018), generate dodgy data, systematically review this research and even conduct systematic reviews of the systematic reviews. Recommendations are repeated over and over, more training, more awareness raising, better communication, while little changes. Returning to Mohamed (2024), who like Jones (2021) demonstrates a keenly critical perspective around her doctoral research, unpacks what can underpin what are inappropriate and accepted academic practices. She scathingly points to the time wasted on learning and reproducing poorly developed ideas to shore up "the importance of misaligned theories" in attempts to showcase "epistemic mastery" (Mohamed 2024 p15).

Questions are asked about how we as researchers, policy makers, practitioners and family carers can work together to address these injustices and engage in critical inquiry to expose hidden forces and processes of interaction, making connections between experiences and consciousness (Pacheco and McConnell 2017). One answer is, of course, to involve people with learning disabilities in research, to work together to decide research priorities, think about what questions we should be asking, co-designing research and ensuring research findings reach appropriate audiences. This will necessarily involve a loosening of research design and ethical parameters and expectations. However, and as I document across this book, this should not be a problem, particularly given the ways in which the rules do not count or are considerably flexed when it comes to the treatment of people with learning disabilities.

Concluding thoughts

It is clear small tweaks in healthcare practices could make a considerable difference to the health and wellbeing of people with learning disabilities. Thoughtful listening, the provision of accessible information, the comprehensive recording of patients with learning disabilities, effective annual health checks and seeing the person as human rather than a diagnosis could transform healthcare services. I object to recommendations that healthcare professionals need training to make these adjustments to their practice. Professionals have lost their way often collectively and need to shake themselves from the slumber involved in ignoring the needs of some patients. I say slumber generously as it is clear these failings can be wilful or deliberate. We saw earlier how medical professionals have a responsibility to oppose human rights abuses and not collude in them. Health and medical education, however, could include content about the lives of people with learning disabilities in the curriculum and, indeed, involve people with learning disabilities in this work. Researchers further have a responsibility to address the limitations in our work and think more critically about this area. We should work with, and for people, and be more courageous in standing up for people's rights and calling out the numerous and enduring violences and violations.

3

LOVE AND RELATIONSHIPS

Introduction

Relationships, intimate, familial, friendships, collegiate or passing acquaintances, form a core part of our lives, health and wellbeing (Carter et al 2021, Wiesel and Bigby 2016). Pets too, as we may forge human–animal bonds that enhance our lives and generate moments of intense love and companionship (Hussein et al 2021, McConnell et al 2019). Relationships can provide sources of sociality, support, pleasure and intimacy. Love is of course important to people with learning disabilities and, to remove any doubt, this has been 'scientifically' proven by Morentin et al (2008) who conducted a love survey in Spain with just under 400 people with learning disabilities.

The right to intimate relationships and marriage are enshrined in human rights frameworks, legislation and policy initiatives, including the international treaty, the United Nations Convention on the Rights of People with Disabilities (UNCRPD) and the 2014 Care Act and *Valuing People* in the United Kingdom. The UNCRPD includes two specific rights, Home and family (Article 23) and Sexual reproductive health (Article 25), which outline how we all have the right to choose our sexual identity, have relationships, make sexual choices and have children (Pérez-Curiel et al 2023). We further have the right to access support and education in these areas.

While rights are promoted and there is an increasing focus on relationships and sexual intimacy (Pérez-Curiel et al 2023), people with learning disabilities are often not allowed to love (Ignagni et al 2016) and their experiences in this area can be overwhelmingly negative (Whittle and Butler 2018). Three chapters into this book, it will likely come as no surprise that people can be obstructed or prohibited from developing their sexuality, forming intimate relationships, from

DOI: 10.4324/9781032644868-3

having children (or losing their children if they do) and, consequently, experience higher levels of loneliness and isolation (Alexandra et al 2018). Indeed, staff and family members can be considered friends suggesting limited wider relationship networks (Merrells et al 2019).

A brief dip back in time demonstrates how efforts to support people with learning disabilities to know more about their sexuality by US educators in the1970s was described as a monumental task in which considerable barriers remained (Kempton and Kahn 1991). The success of any initiative or intervention depended on the consistency of the staff delivering it and clear guidelines:

> Without such guidelines too often one staff member would harshly punish a client for a sexual act, while another would make fun of his behavior, and still a third would look the other way.
>
> *(Kempton and Kahn 1991 p104)*

Over 50 years later, the lack of clear guidelines and staff consistency remains untroubled by any discernible intention to uphold the rights enshrined in the UNCRPD. The increase in focus on supporting the intimate relationships of people with learning disabilities has led to a shift to management rather than lessening of restriction and control (Brown and McCann 2018). As Altermark (2017 p13) argues, the dark past functions "as an imaginary in opposition to which understandings of the present are produced".

A dominant contemporary starting point is that post-institutionalisation marks progress to something better, allowing a metaphorical and implicit 'well done' and lack of critical focus on what people's lives are actually like. Feely (2016 p726) uses similar terminology in arguing the dark past of the sexual suppression of people with learning disabilities in Ireland has not reduced; instead, fears around reproduction have mutated to concern about the wellbeing of children in terms of neglect, abuse or malnutrition. Boundaries between public and private are blurred and the sexuality of people with learning disabilities remains a "heavily gated, deeply moralised and zealously controlled matter" (Bahner et al 2024 p172).

Historic eugenic residues are all too apparent as people with learning disabilities are seen as too naive and childlike *or* too potentially sexually promiscuous to engage with sexual intimacy. Women with learning disabilities are seen as particularly vulnerable while men are allowed more sexual leniency. Contradictions abound which leaves young people, for example, on the cusp of adulthood trapped in what has been described as an 'almost-adult' state in relation to sexual identities (Wilkinson et al 2015). These contradictions include being presented as 'normal' by family carers who concurrently highlight the young person's vulnerability and deficiency (Wilkinson et al 2015). Sexual consent is adaptable and is mostly adapted to remain convenient for non-disabled people (Onstot 2019).

The normative expectation of sexual light touch or no touch in this area further erases consideration of same sex, transgender or non-binary relationships. The assumption is people with learning disabilities *cannot* be LGBTQ+ (Jungels and Bender 2015, Santinele Martino 2017), and almost insurmountable barriers remain. Unsurprisingly, given many of us may remember awkwardness or discomfort when conversations about sexuality or sexual activity were broached within families, discussion of sex between people and family carers can be embarrassing and too easily shut down (Wilkinson et al 2015).

People with profound learning disabilities are further seen to be unable to engage in sexual activity and less likely to have sexual needs, again speaking to assumption-driven practices and the denial of sexual rights (Charitou et al 2021). This seeps into research practice as illustrated by Vehmas' (2019 p521) reflections about his ignorance and associated assumptions in not considering the sexual rights of participants in his research, describing how apart from masturbation, the thought of any further sexual activity is 'an absolute no-no'. Sexual expressions by participants generated feelings of anguish for Vehmas until he recognised these feelings reflected his own discomfort about the thought of profoundly disabled people having sex.

Of course, profoundly disabled people have sexual rights like everyone else and these should not be denied. It is grimly fascinating that among all the philosophical tussling and academic discussion in this area, a good friend who has since died used to leave her profoundly disabled teenage daughter sitting on the toilet alone for some time after recognising that she was trying, and able, to touch her vagina. I would love to share with her the work of Don Kulick (2015) which I return to below.

In this chapter, I explore the intimate relationships and sexual identities of people with learning disabilities and highlight dominant testimonial and hermeneutical epistemic injustices in this area. Indeed, sexual intimacy surfaces eugenic fears in extreme and sometimes absurd ways as people are perceived to be sexually promiscuous or non-sexual, somehow incapable of, too capable of, or uninterested in intimate relationships. Underpinning this is an endorsement and widely held acceptance that intimacy and/or sex-less lives are acceptable for people with learning disabilities. I discuss relationships between people with learning disabilities, family members and paid support staff, unpacking issues around respect, value and the mediation of interpersonal relationships. Pregnancy and parenthood also generate extreme and ungrounded fears which are evidenced by sometimes deceitful and dishonest acts of violence meted out by family courts. Finally, I investigate how people negotiate issues around sexuality, gender and identity, including acts of resistance and subversion, and interactional and symbolic meaning making that offers some hope for change.

Beginning with a brief look back

People with learning disabilities have been prevented from having relationships historically for reasons which do not stand up to much scrutiny. 'Mental deficiency' was held to be synonymous with criminality and sexual promiscuity (Kempton and Kahn 1991); there were eugenic fears around procreation, and people were perceived to be asexual or too vulnerable (Rojas et al 2016). Too this, too that, and too the other. It is extraordinary how nimble, adept and flexible the excuses for why people with learning disabilities cannot do certain things have been and still are. And how empty and meaningless the rhetoric around autonomy, choice and independence actually is.

In many parts of the world, these fears led to brutalising and inhumane measures, including involuntary sterilisation sometimes without people's knowledge, institutionalisation and sexual segregation. The United States led the way in committing to arguably the most extreme of these measures, involuntary sterilisation and there was legislative support for this across numerous states (Amy and Rowlands 2018). The engagement with this programme and embracing of its intentions is illustrated by an excoriating editorial in the *New England Journal of Medicine* published in 1933:

> The burden on society resulting from this increase in feeble-mindedness is tremendous. For one thing, persons with subnormal intelligence are always potential criminals ... The financial loss to the country is appalling. Including both the direct cost of supporting these sufferers from mental disease and the loss of productive capacity due to their incompetence ... the annual total cost of mental disease for the United States [is] around three-quarters of a billion dollars ... We should ... recognize this danger that threatens to replace our population with a race of feeble-minded; we must study its causes and the sources from which it springs. If we wait too long, this viper that we have nourished may prove our undoing.
>
> *(Editorial 1933 p852)*

A year later, the editors wrote in support of the Nazi regime in Germany describing it as "perhaps the most progressive nation in restricting fecundity among the unfit" (Editorial 1934 p.379). The unfit included 'habitual prisoners', people with mental ill health and/or learning disabilities and people who were poor.

Over 30 US states adopted compulsory laws leading to the sterilisation of more than 60,000 people (Suuberg 2020), and 37 states had restrictive marriage statutes (Carey 2009). In 1973, 23 US states still had laws allowing involuntary sterilisation. Only three US states have offered reparations to those affected, the latest being California in 2021.

Other countries, including Japan, Mexico, Canada, New Zealand, Germany, Scandinavia and Switzerland, were close behind. In Canada, between 1928 and 1972, 2,800 cases of involuntary sterilisation of disabled people took place, with most happening in Alberta where the Alberta Sexual Sterilisation Act (1928) aimed to remove sexual practices for this group, poor people and racialised communities (Martino and Perreault-Laird 2019). In the 1920s and 1930s in Aotearoa, New

Zealand, women with learning disabilities were incarcerated and forcibly sterilised (Bloom and Morison 2024). Inmates at the Perttula Institution in Finland were 'alegally' sterilized between 1912 and 1922 as the area sat outside the law (Vehmas and Mietola 2021), while sterilisation and forced abortion was passed in 1938 in Iceland and remained until 1975 (Stefánsdóttir and Hreinsdóttir 2013). Sterilisation continued in Sweden until 1976 (Denekens et al 1999).

Eugenic arguments in favour of sterilisation have been consistent internationally. People with learning disabilities and other marginalised groups sap the strength of the country and generate national concerns about being reproductively swamped with incompetence as alluded to in the editorial extract above (Lee and Morgan 1988, Suuberg 2020). The argument was sometimes framed in a beneficent albeit still brutal way. As Supreme Court Justice Oliver Wendell Holmes in the case of *Buck vs Bell* (1927) stated:

> It is better for all the world if, instead of waiting to execute dangerous degenerate offspring for crimes or to let them starve for their imbecility, society can prevent those who are manifestly unfit from continuing their kind. The principle that sustains compulsory vaccination is broad enough to cover cutting the Fallopian tubes .... Three generations of imbeciles are enough.
>
> *(Paul 1974)*

It was better to prevent people being born than to deal with the fallout of their degenerate presence. There was strong public support for this position as illustrated by a letter published in the *Los Angeles Times* magazine in 1936 with the writer stating their amazement at "right thinking people" letting "imbeciles have children" (Suuberg 2020 p126).

To act as a counterbalance to such disproportionate responses, Eygló Ebba Hreinsdóttir, an Icelandic woman with learning disabilities has talked about how, when she was 27 and living in an institution, a staff member told her she had been sterilised aged 14. She described how:

> After I started to tell my story and talk about the past, I realized it was not my fault and I should not be ashamed. It was not our fault we had to undergo sterilization. It was the government that decided how people with intellectual disabilities were treated. They should be ashamed. People should know that.
>
> *(Stefánsdóttir and Hreinsdóttir 2013 p305)*

Newgenics in the here and now

Eugenic practices have continued into this century, sometimes described as 'newgenics', 'neo-genics' or liberal eugenics (Campbell 2017), that is, less visible mechanisms that continue to restrict the sexual expression of people with learning disabilities (Suuberg 2020). Of course, less visible eugenic mechanisms have always existed, and I outline some in the section below. Research highlights how eugenic practices continue and are seen as acceptable or even important in some countries. Some GPs in Australia, for example, think sterilisation is desirable, particularly for women with learning disabilities (Gilmore and Malcolm 2014), and support workers and family members in New Zealand think it is appropriate under certain conditions (Hamilton 2015).

In Taiwan, sterilisation is encouraged and people with learning disabilities are 'offered', often without consultation subsidised sterilisation costs under the 1984 Taiwan Genetic Health Law (Chou and Lu 2011). Family members offer different explanations in support of the sterilisation of their relative which include removing the work involved in managing menstruation for family members and support workers, the risk of 'chi-fu' (of being taken advantage of) and to reduce the burden on other family members when the mother is no longer able to provide care. Chou and Lu (2011) found participants (parents or partners) were pragmatic in their discussions of 'removing the uterus' to erase these problems. Public health nurses actively intervened in the lives of some participants and one mother was praised when she agreed to the sterilisation of her daughter as she approached puberty.

There is an obvious defiance of logic in these arguments as sterilisation is proposed for people who are deemed to lack capacity, are not able to give informed consent to have intimate relations or are unable to raise a child (Pérez-Curiel et al 2023). The flip side to Justice Holmes's argument about heading off problems through forced sterilisation is that women with learning disabilities are left open to 'consequence free' sexual abuse through an inhumane process presented as in their best interests. The notion that sterilising women will remove the risk of burdensome babies further raises concerns about domestic violence and abuse, particularly in countries such as Taiwan where these issues are considered private (Chou and Lu 2011).

These publicly accepted and endorsed violences again unfold against the background of the UNCPRD. Taiwan, for example, adopted the UNCPRD using domestic mechanisms in 2014; however, the reproductive rights of women with learning disabilities remain ignored (Lu and Beddoe 2023). Countries such as Sweden and the United Kingdom have ratified the UNCRPD while having no national policies, regulations or guidelines to support the development of disabled people's sexuality. These anomalies and absences take us back to the child who was excluded from mainstream school 'because ... the wall bars'.

This peculiar and unfathomable absence and omission creates a void in the lives of people with learning disabilities – an emotional, physical and epistemological void generated by a loose collective of support workers and providers, health and social care professionals, policy makers, politicians and sometimes family carers, who choose not to acknowledge, or actively deny that people with learning disabilities have sexual identities and should be supported to have intimate relationships. Information that supports the views of this collective can be privileged to the extent stories are sought to provide corroborating evidence of, for example, sexual inappropriateness (Perlin and Lynch 2016).

Standardised measures, such as the *Sexuality Knowledge and Awareness Assessment* or the *General Sexual Knowledge Questionnaire* which are designed to perform sexual capacity assessments, can be misused by clinicians to define deviant sexual behaviour on the part of men to prevent sexual intimacy, and are not used with women at all (Thompson et al 2016). The use of sanitised and 'de-sexed' language around sexuality can further downgrade the seriousness of, for example, rape to 'inappropriate behaviour', allowing the continuation of these acts. One person with learning disabilities, in Sirotkin's (2024) examination of Safeguarding Adult Reviews, was able to continue abusing other residents for a decade because the risk of this was not taken seriously because of the language used.

These are serious and substantial issues that remain largely hidden from view and ignored. Perlin and Lynch (2016) suggest (false) "ordinary common sense" prevails which involves people uncritically accepting a position as common-sense practice without making any attempt to deconstruct the logic underpinning it. One example of this is the obstruction of the development of sexual relationships by the argument the minds of people with learning disabilities are comparable to those of children – 'she has a mental age of 3' – which is clearly nonsense. The absence of any scientific or theoretical basis to ordinary common sense is ignored, allowing those with power to lean into chosen stereotypes and consider negative freedoms, in this instance, no sexual relationship, as the only alternative (Onstot 2019).

Supporting positive freedoms could, for example, involve allowing more time and support for people with learning disabilities to learn about sexual intimacy, although there is, again, caution around focusing efforts on educating people with learning disabilities which misattributes responsibility for change rather than addressing the constraints and impoverished opportunities that limit them (Ginn 2022 p930). Instead of a directive and gatekeeping role, support staff should support people's interest in pursuing relationships that may involve some level of risk, as well as helping them to end abusive ones (Bates et al 2017).

'Soft' eugenics

Myriad mechanisms to prevent sexual expression exist beyond sterilisation, segregation and institutionalisation. While reproductive technologies have considerably advanced, the focus among researchers on, for example, genetic inheritance and the development of advanced genetic technologies remains constant (Hashiloni-Dolev et al 2019, Suuberg 2020) and the biological determinism underpinning eugenics remains strong (Proctor 1992).

On perhaps a smaller scale, there remains a lack of easily available, accessible, affirmative resources to support people develop their sexual identities and relationships. People do not know what they do not know, and for people with learning disabilities who are often excluded from the cultural, social, geographical and other spaces in which young people discover and learn about sexual intimacy, this leaves considerable gaps in understanding. The following extract illustrates this exclusion in a series of seemingly mundane statements about the difficulty participants in an Australian study experienced around friendship 'maintenance':

> Grace described the amount she saw her friends, "Well, not that often, in all honesty … Well, because I don't have friends my own age, I don't get to go to parties and to go to that sort of stuff." Jodi also described her infrequent interaction with friends, "I hardly see them," along with John, "I don't see him much these days." Daniel described how interaction with friends depended on program attendance, "Not as much as I used to … Depends. Well, it depends whether …depends if they're doing the same activity as me."
>
> *(Merrells et al 2019 p18)*

Without this knowledge, people are bereft of understanding the basics, let alone intricacies, of negotiating sexual identities, practices or relationships, or engaging with support staff or people close to them about this topic (McCarthy et al 2022, Wilkinson et al 2015). People are effectively denied the right to become socially and sexually competent.

The lack of access to sexual education, to being supported to develop sexual identities and enjoy sexual intimacy is a mechanism that works to ensure people with learning disabilities remain in a sex-less space. However, the lack of information and associated understandings leaves people more vulnerable to sexual abuse. Safeguarding considerations, as we saw in Chapter 1, can be underpinned by ignorance without consideration of current cultural, political, policy and social contexts, and can inhibit discussion about sexual expression (Charitou et al 2021, Wilkinson et al 2015). There is, for example, a lack of safeguarding consideration around forced marriage in the United Kingdom despite women and men with learning disabilities having a five times greater risk of forced marriage than non-disabled people (Clawson et al 2020). Even supposedly robust processes and procedures to protect people can fail them, as evidenced by an estimated 1 in 3 people with learning disabilities experiencing sexual abuse (Tomsa et al 2021).

Abuse rates are higher in residential settings, and one study of reported abuse cases in residential settings in the Netherlands, found staff and people with learning disabilities could be perpetrators. The latter were typically moved instead of addressing the lack of sexual literacy despite evidence this can be effective (Amelink et al 2021). People can fall foul of not knowing and have punitive measures enacted, with sense, kindness and appropriate support absent. Cases of sexual abuse are underreported (Willot et al 2020) and are rarely addressed. Only a small percentage make it to court with around a 1% chance of conviction (Byrne 2018). There is a further knock-on effect that providers can take the lack of police action or failure to prosecute as evidence that nothing happened leading to a lack of internal investigation or scrutiny (Sirotkin 2024).

The information that exists about sexual relationships is dominated by possibilities of disappointment, unwanted pregnancy or abuse (Rushbrooke et al 2014). People are prevented from making errors in judgement in relationships or experiencing the emotionally, even physically, difficult situations that many of us are all too familiar with. As Shelton (1992) suggests, there is a question around how willing staff are to take risks, to allow people the opportunity to experience what most of us will experience across our sexual development.

The call for more information and resources relating to the sexual relationships and rights for people with learning disabilities has been a consistent feature in research for over two decades (see, for example, Christian et al 2001, Rushbrooke et al 2014 and Yool et al 2003). Rights-based information with clear, affirmative and supportive content that includes sex, sexual pleasure and different sexual formats is needed (Whittle and Butler 2018), although this on its own is not enough. Access to pleasure is a human right and it is a serious injustice to discount or override this. Participants in one US-based study described sensuality, arousal and emotional closeness and the associated loneliness experienced as a lack of this (Turner and Crane 2016). Kristy, for example, describes her sexual activity with Duane:

> Well, I like the touching, of his penis. And he gets excited by kissing, passionately. And I said, "we're getting a little excited there, aren't we?" Yeah. We tease each other and I think that's what makes a great relationship.
>
> *(Turner and Crane 2016 p687)*

Alongside the lack of information and education, service providers often lack policies to guide staff in this area. Policy and training that exist again focuses on safety and preventing abuse rather than supporting sexual relationships and promoting sexual rights. Without guidelines, even where there is more leniency, staff may make judgements which inevitably fall back onto their own morals and value judgements or avoid the topic altogether. Parent carers are also given no support to know how to support their children's sexual development as they become adults and there is a question here about whose responsibility this work is or should be.

The avoid or ignore approach has considerable purchase. Some providers in Taiwan declined to take part in a two-year intervention study to improve the quality of life of people with learning disabilities by increasing sexual knowledge and positive attitudes. They expressed concern that the intervention content could encourage people's desire for sexual activities and evoke parental dissent (Chou et al 2020). Staff may only engage with the topic if an issue arises or the person being supported raises it (Charitou et al 2021), and even then, the person can be thwarted, as illustrated by the following extract:

> Because the individual knows that you are a worker and he's not supposed to talk with you in certain ways … we can say that it's not appropriate to do that

> … if it's not directed to you, um … just change the topic, "Oh, have you seen the sun today?"
>
> *(Martino and Perreault-Laird 2019 nd)*

In instances where people with learning disabilities bring up sexual activity, the response has been described as if the "resident has made a profane affront to the moral order" (Bahner et al 2024 p169). The strength of this response suggests a phobic reaction; the idea of people with learning disabilities having intimate relationships is revolting.

The encouraged approach to 'redirect' the conversation is demeaning, disrespectful and works to silence expression. The complex exercising of power through these non- or negative responses will likely impact how people with learning disabilities view sexual practices. Indeed, silence conveys a negative meaning and is a form of management by non-recognition. That is, people with learning disabilities are constructed as non-sexual (Shildrick 2007). There is no freedom or opportunity to discuss sexual expression as permissible conversations are firmly adjudicated by staff and family members (Martino and Perreault-Laird 2019). Reproducing regulation around what are considered to be acceptable conversations allows the denial of sexuality and sexual rights to continue.

In Sweden, the sexuality of people with learning disabilities is largely ignored with an approach underpinned by the logic if nothing happens then nothing can go wrong (Bahner et al 2024). Ignoring is not benign, however, as staff actively work to ensure there is no sexual intimacy among or between the people they support. Subtle indications of power are particularly present in relation to considerations of sexual intimacy. Kulick's (2015) work comparing the sexual lives of disabled people in Sweden and Denmark was prompted by hearing about a disabled Swedish woman who finally experienced orgasms when her male support workers lifted her into the bath. Once staff realised what was happening, they stopped doing it. Danish support staff recognise their role in supporting people's erotic desires; there are national guidelines around supporting people to engage with their sexuality and an accredited course exists to become a sexual advisor. The guidelines prohibit sexual relationships between the person being supported and their support worker, though they can be supported to learn to masturbate and engage with sex workers. Danish guidelines present the responsibility of the support worker in the following terms:

> A helper should be aware that he or she should be able to counsel and support an individual in relation to sexuality. However, a helper may not be ordered by his or her workplace to help an individual learn to practice sex. If a person needs assistance to practice sex, then the helper, however, does have the duty to see to it that another helper or a qualified expert is referred to that person.
>
> *(Kulick 2015 pS244)*

The 'ignore and hope it goes away' approach to sexuality is, likely, widespread despite the Danish example of upholding people's sexual rights, and whilst we see resistance from some people with learning disabilities, sometimes with the tacit support of staff which I return to below, it is too easy to ignore or dismiss this issue.

In more practical terms, there can be a lack of staff to facilitate meeting other people, a lack of social opportunities, and staff shift patterns may finish earlier than social events further curtailing social lives. Providers can actively discourage consideration of sexuality with explicit instructions given in staff training to avoid the subject of sexuality which can leave staff feeling further compromised, vulnerable and uncomfortable (Deffew et al 2022).

Other mechanisms of soft eugenics include provider rules that inhibit privacy, such as not being allowed to have overnight guests, the prohibition of expressions of affection like holding hands or always having to have bedrooms doors open. There can even be policies that restrict flirting within segregated spaces, described by Turner and Crane (2016) as paternalistic and punitive. Some people share bedrooms meaning even less privacy and small group homes can be sex-segregated without consideration of same-sex relationships (Santinele Martino 2022). As Tatiana said,

> I'm looking for a boyfriend. It's not allowed to be any boyfriend from workshop [one of the workshop rules] … only [out in the] community
>
> *(Santineli Martino 2022 p1234)*

Preventing relationships within segregated spaces can have considerable impact on people's social lives as opportunities to go to different places and meet people are often absent. One participant commented on their wish for more privacy, where sex could be "more than just five or ten minutes, people rush here because there are people around" (McCarthy 1997 p117). Staff disrupted relationships between people with learning disabilities by bringing along other people without agreement, explicitly demonstrating disrespect (Robinson and Idle 2023). A Swedish study found constrained sexual scripting for people living in care settings both in post-institutionalised settings and the wider community (Bahner et al 2024). The authors argue there is a pressing need to empower people with learning disabilities to express their sexuality within the context of sexual rights.

Surveillance techniques of control are substantial and seamlessly breach boundaries reaching beyond where the person lives to data exchanges between homes, public transport operators, the police and members of the public. In Ireland, the decline in the influence of the Catholic Church after the disclosure of widespread historical sexual abuse practices has led to social workers and other professionals policing sexuality, and a shift to a secular discourse around what are appropriate behaviours (Feely 2016). People with learning disabilities continue to be denied opportunities to develop intimate relationships because sexual expression remains considered inappropriate behaviour.

Focusing on a day centre service in Ireland he calls Rathberg, Feely (2016) draws on the work of Deleuze and Foucault to create the Rathberg sexual surveillance assemblage, examining how material and discursive elements affect the stories told. In one example, two women were "caught snogging the heads off each other" in the gym hot tub on CCTV (Feely 2016 p732). While in another, a man with learning disabilities was removed from the day centre because of a developing relationship. For Feely, the material elements in these examples include space, information technologies and visceral affects, while discursive elements include provider rules, attitudes and psychiatric discourses of normality and abnormality. This analysis lays bare stark surveillance practices that operate to prohibit sexual relationships, drawing on interweaving discourses and actors which include parents, providers, public, judgements around 'levels' of learning disabilities, the alarm flag of statutory rape and ubiquitous safeguarding. Feely (2016 p747) describes the "soft power of the disability service" where "the rules are made up on a thoroughly ad hoc basis". There is no sense or reason behind these rules and yet they remain unchallenged or overlooked because of the pervasiveness of ordinary common sense (Perlin and Lynch 2016) and the associated removal of any owning of, or allocating, responsibility.

Conundrums, fear and uncertainties

Recent research has focused on the role of support workers in facilitating or otherwise the sexual expression of people they work with. Stepping outside of the enlightened and comprehensive approach in Denmark, this literature highlights conflicts, contradictions and the ambivalence support workers can experience around this area (Deffew et al 2022). Support workers are gatekeepers of knowledge, with power and influence over what the people they support could, should or should not know or can or cannot do. In effect, they can uphold basic human rights in decision making, and promote, ignore or prohibit people's sexual expression (Bloom and Morison 2024, McCarthy et al 2022). For Löfgren-Mårtenson (2004, p.197), they are the 'institutional walls' supporting formal policies restricting, for example, women's sexuality.

Staff actions can be stymied, however, by the sometimes-inexplicable rules of their employers described above, the lack of support and guidance in this area and austerity burdened social care contexts. Safety trumps the promotion of sexual rights and agency, captured here by a support worker in Northern Ireland:

> I'm sitting here and I feel like a complete hypocrite, because there is so much that I would love to be able to do but my hands are tied. If they [the clients] came to me and asked me for help I couldn't do it because my job and my neck would be on the line.
>
> *(Lafferty et al 2012 p35)*

Over a decade later, an extract from another support worker in New Zealand presents the baked in ambivalence, contradiction and eugenic undertones that dominate this area:

> It's a really hard area to talk about, because some people might be feeling that people with intellectual disability shouldn't have any sexual interactions. … I don't know how we support them, because we don't know how much they understand and how much we should go for it, push to talk. So, it's quite [a] hard topic. [laughs] […] [pause] If I gave that information, it could be too much and they might be overwhelmed, and they could go to the extreme outside of this. We don't know how much they are really, fully understanding. […] Yeah, confusion, and, I don't know … probably, they could be too curious if we give a lot of information. It is just a really hard one [laughs].
>
> *(Bloom and Morison 2024 p406)*

Some of what is captured in this extract reminds me of the Taiwanese provider mentioned earlier who did not want to encourage thoughts around sexual intimacy. The argument that any discussion around sexual intimacy would encourage curiosity and that 'they could go to the extreme outside of this' underlines the lingering stain of historic discourses around control and sexual promiscuity. And yet, given these discussions are not had, how can support staff possibly know? These prejudicial statements and the phobic responses underpinning them, openly expressed within the context of a research interview, are revealing and concerning.

The often-wholesale erasure of consideration of sexuality on the part of staff is apparent and consistent across many high-income countries. One social worker in an Israeli study described how many of the people with learning disabilities have no interest in sex and intimacy, they are too 'low-functioning' to become aroused and it's not relevant to them (Holler and Bondorevsky-Heyman 2023 p826). An English study using vignettes to explore the sexual experiences of people with learning disabilities found staff members were unsure of their role in this context as they had no experience of it. One participant described how they could count the times on one hand when they had to deal with a conversation or 'behaviour' about sex (Maguire et al 2019 p62). A participant in an Irish study, seemingly prompted by the research questions, reported being shocked they had never seen intimate relationships mentioned in care plans (Deffew et al 2022 p1054). References to sexual intimacy where they existed were likely to be included in behavioural support plans and categorised as negative behaviour.

The absence or denial of consideration of sexual expression is accompanied by inherently disrespectful, infantilising and dismissive language. For example, Grace said:

> Um, we have sleepovers, we play in the pool, we play in the park, just bits and pieces, depends what we feel like on the day.
>
> *(Merrells et al 2019 p17)*

Examples from studies in Sweden, England and New Zealand demonstrate similar techniques of infantilisation and the use of similar terminology:

> The residents are like brothers and sisters.
>
> *(Bahner et al 2024 p169)*

> They might peck each other on the lips but no more than that. (Participant 4)
>
> They just meet up at their local disco, sit and chat, hold hands have a dance then we go home [laughs] nothing really, yeah that's about it. (Participant 3)
>
> *(Maguire et al 2019 p62)*

> As I said, these ones here, I haven't seen that with them. I haven't seen anything like kissing. … One of the girls will give the boys a peck, but she does that to everyone, or she tells you that she loves them and that sort of thing but there's no. … I don't read anything else into it.
>
> *(Bloom and Morison 2024 p404)*

It is difficult to read these extracts over two decades after the publication of *Valuing People* in England which presented such strong statements about the importance of autonomy and independence for people with learning disabilities. You have control over your life, but we are going to treat you like a child forever. A forever child, in a homogenous group of forever children with a peck on the cheek on a playdate.

Frustration about the lack of change is apparent in some published research. Deffew et al (2022) found little change for staff supporting people with learning disabilities in relation to sexuality and relationships over a decade. They state a marker needs to be laid down to ensure the same observations are not being made in another 10 years:

> As a fundamental human right, people with an intellectual disability are required to have the ability to express their sexuality freely. It is, therefore, essential that service providers and staff aid them in fulfilling this right. It is with this understanding that this research is a call to action; it is a call for change.
>
> *(Deffew et al 2022 p1057)*

Laying down markers and calls to action that feature in more activist-orientated research are important, though can remain unheeded, as we saw in Chapter 2 with Popay's call for the public health community to speak up against social injustices. I return to this point in Chapter 5.

As well as ambivalence, the hesitancy or fear support workers express around even talking about the sexual expression of the people they support is striking. Fear creates cautious actions in relation to sexual expression and underlines how support workers themselves are bound by power relations. While they may be able to exercise power over the people they support, they are in turn caught up in other power struggles, particularly given support work itself reflects gendered, racialised and classed asymmetries of care work (Munévar 2021). It is a pressured, precarious and poorly renumerated occupation generating "debilitating landscapes of care" (MacPherson et al 2023 p140) which is not conducive to the sensitive and careful support people need to develop their sexual identities. High staff turnover and precarious employment, including temporary or agency labour can further lead to cursory engagement with people's lives, aspirations and desires by staff, and a focus on the key indicators prioritised by providers and regulatory processes (Sirotkin 2024). Staff are forced to negotiate a complex ethical landscape with multiple competing demands, including the service culture and restrictions, family members and fear and anxiety about potential risks (Santinele Martino 2022).

Family members can play a key role in supporting or inhibiting the sexual development of people with learning disabilities (Charitou et al 2021, Rojas et al 2016). Some parents support their children in this area (Kulick 2015, Rose 2023). For example, in Brazil, parents were found to be supportive of intimate relationships in the future, although there was uncertainty and concern about risks of promiscuity and the importance of support and clear guidelines (Monteiro et al 2023). Other parents exercise considerable and unchallenged power in preventing opportunities for relationships, including controlling contraception use (Rose 2023). Ginette Green (aged 19 years) spoke about her relationship with Simon:

> I have a boyfriend; his name is Simon and he calls me his girlfriend. I see him sometimes. I don't call him up on the phone because Mum says I'm not allowed to, so I use Facebook. Sometimes he comes on my Facebook, talks to me online. I said, "How are you?" and he said, "I'm fine". He is friendly and good-looking and a nice person.
>
> *(O'Shea and Frawley 2020 p661)*

One participant in a Canadian study described how his mother allowed him to masturbate in his bedroom, but he was not allowed to have a relationship or engage in other sexual acts such as watching pornography (Santineli Martino 2022). Our *Flourishing Lives* study found parent participants wanted their children to have 'someone to cuddle' though shied away from seriously considering intimate relationships (Ryan and O'Brien 2024). Daniel, a research participant in a Swedish study, said:

> It was [my girlfriend's] mother who thought that she wouldn't be able to take care of a child. She has Asperger's, so...
>
> Interviewer: But it's your right to decide ...
>
> Yes, but her mother decided a lot. [My girlfriend] got sterilized.
>
> *(Bahner et al 2024 p170)*

Gender and sexuality

Research suggests romantic relationships can be particularly important for women as they can help them understand their gender, and aspirations as girlfriend, fiancé, wife and mother (O'Shea and Frawley 2020), positions which are 'normal' (Bates et al 2017) and show women with learning disabilities are desirable and lovable. Post-institutionalisation, however, has not removed or reduced the risk of sexual abuse that women, in particular, experience (McCarthy 1997, Wiseman and Ferrie 2020), not least because of the enduring lack of information, resources and support around sexuality (Rose 2023). Women continue to experience sexual and reproductive regulation (Bloom and Morison 2024). In one Safeguarding Adult Review in England, for example, a woman with learning disabilities was dressed in 'high tight knickers' and locked in her room to keep men away from her. A case conference was suggested to establish if her behaviour was making her more vulnerable to men (Sirotkin 2024).

Men with learning disabilities are granted more opportunities to have sexual relations than women who are often seen to have diminished or no sexual desires, as vulnerable and in need of protection (Bloom and Morison 2024, Vehmas 2019), or immoral, vulnerable and dangerous (AM 2022). Men with or without learning disabilities are granted more opportunities to have sexual relations with women with learning disabilities through the combined practices of a lack of information, infantilisation, forced contraception and silencing of the topic of sexuality.

Forced precautionary contraception is common with contraceptive implant the most used form as decided by family caregivers or support staff (Wickström et al 2020). We saw earlier how this practice eases the work of caregivers, and it is easier to manage menstruation through medication than it is to produce accessible information and support for women with learning disabilities, family members and support workers. There can be resistance on the part of family members in this area to engaging with bodily and material aspects of menstruation (Goli et al 2020).

An alternative approach to the menstruation of women with profound learning disabilities can be found in a study of frontline workers in institutional settings in Taiwan where staff used menstruation as a way of checking women's health and as a form of communication (Chen et al 2022). The exploration of the cultural paradox of care in this study, which involved dignity and hierarchies, demonstrates how people with learning disabilities were still infantilised and staff commitment to Confucian care ethics was exploited.

In India, marriage possibilities discussed in relation to men are not extended to women because of fears sexual abuse will be legitimised and hidden by marriage (AM 2022). These fears are reflected elsewhere (see, for example, Barger et al 2009, Pan and Ye 2012). We saw earlier how barriers to the development of intimate relationships can facilitate the perpetuation of forced marriages and abuse of people with learning disabilities. Opposition to marriage remains largely consistent although some parents would like their daughter or son to get married for peace of mind (McCarthy et al 2022, Taghizadeh et al 2020) or because of a belief that marriage will cure the impairment (Pérez-Curiel et al 2023).

Heteronormative and cisnormative attitudes of family members, health professionals and other people with learning disabilities can dominate this area with further risks that gender identity is perceived as an example of behavioural issues (Abbott 2015). There is little or no accessible information or resources to support gender diverse young people with learning disabilities develop their sexual identities, and the experiences of transgender people with learning disabilities are almost invisible (Smith et al 2022).

A review of the social inclusion of LGBTQ+ and gender diverse adults in learning disabilities services included nine papers from the United Kingdom, USA, Iceland, and Netherlands (Smith et al 2022). Of these, only three included transgender people who experienced extreme pressure to comply with cisgender expectations. The lack of staff confidence, knowledge and ability to support LGBTQ+ and gender diverse adults was magnified. The routes for some heterosexual people with learning disabilities to access support was denied to those who sat outside of gender normativity and providers offered no support to staff in this area. Indeed, support workers in an Irish study were emphatic that LGBTQ+ relationships would never happen, and the topic was too sensitive for their service (Deffew et al 2022).

People can, understandably, be fearful of coming out to support staff, family members or others. It is hard to come out even when you have the resources, tools and cultural references to do so, and there can be a fear of acceptance, or belief that your parents or others would not approve. There is evidence that people with learning disabilities can be negative, or that people experience wider abuse and prejudice, and yet, once again, a big leap is not needed to support people to feel accepted, as Charlie who attended a LGBTQ support group in a secure learning disability unit describes:

> they welcomed us, like, when we first went, they said hello to us and asked me my name, and they introduced themselves, and I just really, really liked it. . .I felt safer at the group, cos the people there are like, like I said, like me.
>
> *(Tallentire et al 2020 p22)*

Wilkinson et al (2015), like Deffew et al (2022), found similar stigmatising attitudes remained from a decade before and having learning disabilities created a 'double disadvantage' in developing LGBTQ+ sexual identities. Gary, for example, said:

> I do think I was gay at school, 'cause I liked guys, I didn't like girls mostly. Well, then I decided not to be gay, cause I got bullied. I didn't want to be anything I knew I'd get bullied badly for.
>
> *(Wilkinson et al 2015 p101)*

Evidence suggests relationships and sexual education benefit young people with learning disabilities, as they can increase self-esteem and support decision making around sexuality (McCann et al 2019). It is clear, however, that rights of LGBTQ+ people with learning disabilities remain unsupported and largely abandoned.

Pregnancy and parenthood

Turning to a consideration of pregnancy and parenthood generates further bleakness and the identification of cruelty and phobic practices. Pregnancy is typically viewed as problematic for people with learning disabilities. It is something to be avoided or not considered an option. Lingering eugenic assumptions link learning disability with genetic flaws, and reproduction can be disavowed (Turner and Crane 2016). Article 23 of the UNCRPD states every effort should be made to keep the family unit intact and yet parents with learning disabilities trigger anxiety (Callow et al 2017) and, as I illustrate below, extreme and unjust actions.

These discourses can be deeply felt. People with learning disabilities may think they are not fit to be parents or are persuaded by staff they are not able to bring up children. The threat of child removal can loom large and the strength of these ableist normative positions is hard to resist from a position of epistemic and pragmatic powerlessness:

> Well, babies are hard to bring up, see. They're very hard to bring up on your own. Cause I'm a handicapped, and if something happened to the baby, say I tried to go like that [jerks her head to one side] or something like that, I might drop the baby and I don't want to drop the baby, in one sense, in one way. So I said to my friend, I haven't told the doctor or the nurses yet, I would like to have a, I'd like, what is that, abortion. You know, have all the womb out and that like. (21 year old participant)
>
> *(Aull Davies 2007 np)*

At the same time, the strength and importance of motherhood is clear despite the common loss of children:

> Being a mother was always something that I wanted. Something that I dreamed about. No matter if I don't see them every day; I am still Mary and Manuel's mother. I am always their mother (Maria).
>
> *(Pacheco and McConnell 2017 p506)*

A lack of poor or inadequate support and information leads to less informed pregnancies and childbirth, and women with learning disabilities often have caesarian deliveries (Kassee et al 2023, Pérez-Curiel et al 2023), sometimes without being told why (Malouf et al 2017). Parents with learning disabilities report feeling unfairly treated, powerless and unsupported (Sheerin et al 2013). Women can be treated differently to other pregnant woman and mothers by maternity services, as Lisa described:

> I hate being treated differently so like all through my appointments and on the ward I'd been watching how they respond to other people, and how they'd respond to other people was completely different to how they responded to me.
>
> *(Malouf et al 2017 np)*

Lisa also talked about the surveillance she felt she was subjected to once her baby was born.

> We weren't allowed to do anything unless the midwife was supervising us…I felt too nervous to enjoy it…like when you bottle-feed and you just have this odd glance at your husband, or someone who knows it's a proud moment and I just found I had to fix my eyes on my son…I didn't feel I could look somewhere else in case I got marked down for it.
>
> *(Malouf et al 2017 np)*

This surveillance can be particularly disconcerting and intimidating given the lack of support, accessible information and subsequent feelings of ignorance and ill-preparedness. While some mothers in this study felt well supported by antenatal and intrapartum care, others had not been told about parenting classes and described feeling confused after rushed appointments and a lack of accessible information.

Positive aspects of parenthood including love, self-esteem and parental identities are again absent from information with a focus on contraception rather than reproductive planning and support (Tarasoff et al 2020). There is little will or imagination to imagine people with learning disabilities as parents (Höglund et al 2013). Indeed, a systematic review about sexuality and sexual identity found two of the four studies on the topic of parenthood were about pregnancy as an outcome of sexual abuse (Pérez-Curiel et al 2023).

This negativity around potential parenthood is apparent in various countries including Ireland (Feely 2016), Australia (Collings et al. 2018) and Poland (Ćwirynkało and Parchomiuk 2017). In the Netherlands, the government commissioned a mixed methods study into 'good-enough' parenting among people with learning disabilities, with a view to discouraging parenthood among this group. The findings showed that around half the cases were not good-enough parenting, while 33% were good enough and 16% considered doubtful by caregivers (Willems et al 2007). The authors recommend further investigation into contributory factors and more support for parents. It is clear 'the presence of old ideas' continues to inhibit the intimate relationships of people with learning disabilities.

People with learning disabilities are disproportionately likely to have their children removed, leading to experiences of intense grief and loss (Mayes and Llewellyn 2012). There is often little return from the point of removal despite evidence that with early support people are able to look after their children (Malouf et al 2017, Mays and Llewellyn 2012). Indeed, strategies to support pregnant women with learning disabilities include building a relationship with the woman, not questioning the pregnancy or desire for the woman to become a mother, being positive while acknowledging there may be additional needs, offering longer appointments, using clear and accessible language and information and providing women with practical skills (Pérez-Curiel et al 2023).

In the United States, 37 states and four territories allow for the termination of parental rights due to disability, particularly learning disabilities and once involved in child protection processes, 40% of children with a parent with learning disabilities will no longer live with their biological parents (Kendrick 2024). The termination of parental rights is termed the 'civil death penalty' as it kills the legal relationship between parents and a child (Callow et al 2017) generating another form of social murder.

There is contradictory evidence about the risk factors associated with parents with learning disabilities which can include poverty, mental ill health, domestic violence and level of support (Powell et al 2017). An analysis of national level US data from the child protection system found children of parents with learning disabilities were more likely to experience emotional and psychological rather than physical abuse and it is argued being a mother with learning disabilities is a risk indicator rather than risk factor for child maltreatment (Slayter and Jensen 2019). Indeed, the US Federal Departments of Justice and Health and Human Services addressed the issue of parenting and learning disabilities in 2015 with two documents. The second, more technical document includes sensible statements such as:

> if a child welfare agency provides classes on feeding and bathing children and a mother with an intellectual disability needs a different method of instruction to learn the techniques, the agency should provide the mother with the method of teaching that she needs…a child welfare agency should provide the family of the child with the services necessary for the safe return of the child to the child's home in a manner that meets the unique needs of the family.
>
> *(US Department of Justice and US Department of Health and Human Services (2015 pp6–7)*

Despite guidance like this, a set of invisible calculations seem to be made in relation to people with learning disabilities which are not carried out in relation to non-disabled people. These calculations are made without concession to reasonable adjustments or engagement with evidence, and with the odds already stacked against people due to the lack of steps taken to support or inform them. People are effectively set up to fail and penalised accordingly. For Rojas et al (2016 p59), these demands are rarely considered by non-disabled people; we need to think about how some people spend their lives being forced to be part of an unattainable standard and what this means for us all.

I suggest it is worse than trying to force people to be part of an unattainable standard, although in some respects it is difficult to know what is happening because of the distorted scholarship and dodgy data. Indeed, Callow et al (2017), in an analysis of 42 appellate cases involving the termination of parental rights and learning disability, found the term 'evidence based' was not used in any of the proceedings despite the requirement under US laws for courts to consider the scientific basis of evidence presented.

In a similar way to the misuse (abuse) of sexual capacity measures discussed earlier, a close examination of what we know about the area of family courts reveals abhorrent practices and hermeneutical injustice. There is a reliance on IQ testing which we know is not a scientific measure and furthermore does not predict parenting success (Callow et al 2017). The concept of good-enough parenting is not extended to mothers with learning disabilities who are presumed to be incompetent (Pacheco et al 2024). Mothers with learning disabilities are less likely to be offered access to case management services within child protection systems, suggesting less focus on or importance attached to family reunification. There is a lower use of family preservation services and discrepancies between referrals to substance abuse services. In one Canadian study, the authors were unsure if there was a lack of inclusive services, or if the lack of referrals indicated that perceived problems could not be remediated (Pacheco et al 2022). A critical discourse analysis of Quebec family court documents found family members were discredited if they disagreed with the court:

> It is evident the testimony of the mother and grandmother do not correlate with that of the department of youth justice and therefore, little credibility can be given to their position. (Report 6, para 7)
>
> *(Pacheco et al 2024 p329)*

This testimonial injustice is similar to the coronial experiences of families discussed in Chapter 2 where coroners prioritised 'expert' witnesses over the knowledge of family members. Mothers were also rendered voiceless within these court documents although it was not clear how this came about.

An analysis of reports of custody deprivation cases in Iceland similarly found IQ was used as a fluctuating and unscientific master narrative that lacked definitional precision (Sigurjónsdóttir and Rice 2017). This analysis demonstrated how the decision to remove children was made early on in each case and the authors suggest the lack of precision may reflect this. That is, the tools could be used to support an already-made decision. In addition, descriptors such as 'very', 'extremely', 'significantly', and 'much' were used to intensify and worsen the negative content of the report, and documents stated available support and interventions had not been effective when they had not been offered.

These are, again, outlandish findings. The authors conclude a form of diagnostic (or IQ) overshadowing leads to a lack of engagement with the characteristics of the parents. In effect, these cases are measured using cultural knowledge systems which are presented as scientific or perceived to be ordinary common sense. This represents a significant dereliction of duty on the part of senior officials. In a wider Icelandic study, Rice and Sigurjónsdóttir (2018) describe these findings as absurd and interpret the prejudicial treatment parents with learning disabilities experience in the child protection services as a form of structural violence.

These examples provide clear evidence of how professionals and a wider collective act to maintain barriers to parenting by people with learning disabilities, engaging in work which, while possibly presented as well-meaning, is characterised by ignorance, deceit and dishonesty. The embedded prejudices that underpin this labour can be extreme and may constitute phobic responses. I argued in Chapter 1 how learning disability is an obscurely defined and under-examined label and yet responses to it, even within court proceedings, are deployed with remarkable consistency and detrimental effect to people so labelled. I use the idea of a loose (and sometimes shifting) collective here as a heuristic device because so much of what I have presented in this book defies explanation or sense. There is a collective of disparate and diverse social actors whose professional practice, interests, values and actions work across different fields to limit the life opportunities of people with learning disabilities. We could extend Goffman's conceptualisation and term this collective the 'unwise', though this may suggest more coherence than is warranted. And even the wise can fall among the collective in certain contexts such as supporting sexual relationships and identities. Identifying the collective as something that needs addressing is probably as far as we can go here.

What we do know, however, is little or no attempt is made to ensure people are supported in their parenting and there is a wilful refusal to understand and recognise people with learning disabilities are human, have desires and want to, and have the right to, become parents.

Resistance

Despite the considerable efforts to obstruct and prevent sexual expression and intimacy outlined above, people with learning disabilities found ways around this in institutional settings and still do. In the Brandon Training School discussed in Chapter 1, evidence was found of inmates' tenacity in pursuing sex and intimacy that ranged from "undesirable nocturnal activities" to lifelong companionate bonds (Allen and Fuller 2016 np).

Homosexuality was common in US institutions in the mid-20 century (Kempton and Kahn 1991) and post institutionalisation people are taking risks to enjoy sexual relationships in public places such as the forest or parks (Santineli Martino 2022). Feely (2016) found support staff sometimes ignored sexual expressions between people although this could entail risks for them. He suggests people with learning disabilities and staff members demonstrated courage in resisting these surveillance practices, poignantly describing how:

> Jenny's story reminds us again of the risks of resistance but also that staff will, at times, take these risks, creating blind spots, albeit temporary, in the panoptical gaze – thus allowing service users rare opportunities to hold hands, or perhaps to kiss, someone they love.
>
> *(Feely 2016 p744)*

One example of a blind spot was the dimmed quiet room in Rathberg which was used by some people to make out. Feely found participants were able to use these spaces to expand their understanding and reference of what sexuality involves.

Other studies similarly found people with learning disabilities appropriating service provision associated spaces such as day centres for sexual activity or experimentation (Santineli Martino 2022), in effect, doing the ordinary in extraordinary conditions. Some people use the internet, communicating with partners via Facebook as they are not allowed to meet in other ways (O'Shea and Frawley 2020), or as a way of getting to know partners before meeting in real life. People also kept their relationships or sexuality secret from family members or support staff. Mandy, who was engaged to be married described how her mother refused to accept the engagement, and insisted on calling her engagement ring a friendship ring and her fiancé, her boyfriend (O'Shea and Frawley 2020). Mandy created a new subject position of 'slightly engaged' to resist her mother's denial of her relationship.

There are examples of 'the wise', family members or support staff, who are supportive around intimate relationships and provide a good ear to listen to people's concerns or desires. Staff can actively support people around sexual relations by offering advice, sexual education and helping them widen their circle of friends to meet potential partners (Charitou et al 2021). Other examples of resistance include staff at a Keralan rehabilitation centre who supported one attendee to dress up as 'Bharat Mata' the ideal women at a fancy-dress competition. The incredulity this initially generated soon turned to applause (AM 2022). In the same study, a participant was able to partially express her sexual identity by repeatedly calling a man she liked, her cousin-brother despite being teased or ignored by staff and her parents.

Research involving people with learning disabilities offers insights into how the restrictive regulatory silencing around sexual expression can be felt (Bahner et al 2024, Feely 2016). Laura, for example, explained to a researcher, who had been 'warned' by a staff member that she could develop an interest in staff members, that:

> There is something that everybody here knows about, but no one wants to talk about. It's kind of a little open secret here. I do not know if you've been told this

> already, but it was like this: I fell a little bit in love with one of the staff who used to work here, and obviously it ended with him not being allowed to work here anymore. Because that's the way it usually goes. It's one of those things that no one here wants to talk about ... As soon as I bring it up everyone tries to change the topic of conversation, because it's kind of taboo to talk about. I personally think that the staff reckons my feelings will disappear by not talking about it. But that's not really how it works.
>
> *(Bahner et al 2024 p168)*

This acknowledgement of sexual expression being an open secret, and a taboo topic underlines the ableist silencing of the sexuality of people with learning disabilities and the absurdity of staff actions. As Laura says, not talking about something does not make it go away. Strategies of silencing, of removal, of not wanting to encourage sexual desires, or pretending something does not exist are contemporary manifestations of historic eugenic practices and, in the process, reveal so much about the commonly held perceptions about people with learning disabilities.

People also advocate for their freedom and right to privacy and engage in forms of activism to change attitudes (Fulford and Cobingo 2018). Cassandra, for example, was reluctant to tell her father she was bisexual because he already struggled with her disabled identity, and she did not want to reawaken any underlying resentment with a further non-normative identity (Bahner et al 2023). In the same study, Stella, who was struggling to move in with her boyfriend because his limited guardian would not allow it, made sure the people she lived with were aware of their sexual rights. Daniel resorted to lying about what underwear he was wearing, recognising his parents were probably too old to try to understand his choice of clothing.

Parents with learning disabilities also fight back against the removal of their children. In Iceland, parents have been described as strategically surrounding themselves with 'secret weapons' in the form of allies and drawing on human rights protections (Stefánsdóttir et al 2023). Rose (2023) found counter narratives as some participants with learning disabilities in England strongly argued they could be good parents with appropriate support and mothers can resist the way they are perceived by holding on to their valued self and social identities as mothers (Pacheco and McConnell 2017).

What needs to change in a space where so much is so wrong?

Through a systematic review and critical appraisal of the research recommendations of papers about sexuality and intimate relations published between 1972 and 2018, Ginn (2022) is firm in her conclusion that the focus should be on addressing the constraining forces that limit the lives of people with learning disabilities rather than trying to improve people's knowledge and self-efficacy. The weight and volume of recommendations relating to the management of people with learning disabilities is concerning. Ginn (2022) advocates for a groundwork of sufficiently funded rights-based legislation that will enable the creation of effective policies and ensure sanctioning, and resources are available to support staff to make sure people have opportunities for sexual intimacy and relationships.

These conditions would involve support and skill development around emotional and sexual intimacy that includes pleasure, joy and arousal as well as vulnerability, risk-taking and choosing to be known by others. The replication of national or regional guidelines along the lines of those in Denmark, or the Australian state of New South Wales which has a disability policy with clear guidelines for professionals to ensure sexual rights are upheld, including specific support and resources (Bahner 2020), in other countries could support upholding Articles 23 and 25 of the UNCRPD. Some countries, such as Spain and the Netherlands, have sexual assistance initiatives; however, these are not embedded into national policy and can be ambiguous (Bahner et al 2023). It is important to note how precarious and sometimes short-lived any improvements made can be. Examples of this roll back are scattered across this book and in this chapter, Kulick (2015) reported the national guidelines around sexual support he drew on in his study were pared back in the 2012 handbook which superseded them.

Further recommendations to better support relationships and sexuality include support workers, social workers and family members assuming the role of allies (Lu and Beddoe 2023, Rose 2023,Vincent et al 2024); awareness around the impact of service provision change on social networks with ameliorative steps taken to restore these relationships or support people to make new ones; emotional support to help people with the loss of previous relationships (Sullivan et al 2016); self-advocacy led training courses; partnership working between schools, families and providers (Lafferty et al 2012); parenting information and classes; clear information and resources to help people manage child removal (Rose 2023); more privacy including the options to have partners to stay over; and greater visibility and representation of parenting with learning disabilities. As people are more susceptible to abusive relationships or ignorance around areas of birth control or sexual health, they should receive more information and support to form consensual and loving relationships, rather than a closing down of this area:

> Professionals must acknowledge the legitimacy of pleasure for adults with ID [intellectual disability] and, most importantly, create the bridges that will provide access to these meaningful experiences.
>
> *(Turner and Crane 2016 p693)*

These recommendations, alongside many others, highlight differences in power between people, family and paid support workers, and how the 'wins' of the disability movement over decades have barely grazed the lives of people with learning disabilities. While this chapter offers articulation of the subversiveness, courage and resilience of some people with learning disabilities and support staff, the focus on sexual intimacy and reproduction reveals the perniciousness of eugenic thinking. We have more, and repeated, recommendations in this area including sufficiently funded rights-based legislation and resources. Until people with learning disabilities are recognised as human, as people who have rights that should be upheld as part of a just society, by the various and shifting members of the collective, nothing will change.

4

HOME LIFE, HOUSING, COMMUNITY AND EMPLOYMENT

Introduction

Housing is an internationally recognised major determinant of health (Capasso and D'Alessandro 2021, Emerson and Hatton 2014, Martin et al 2011). Where we live, in what kind, size and quality of home or dwelling, with whom and under what type of agreement – ownership, tenancy or other arrangement – is key to our wellbeing (Howden-Chapman et al 2002, Marı'-Dell'Olmo et al 2017). Indeed, home-making and the experience of being at home contributes to our humanity and how others perceive us (Annison 2000). Home is a place that should offer ontological security and freedom from surveillance, and has been described as:

> an emotional warehouse wherein grief, anger, love, regret and guilt are experienced as powerfully real and, at the same time, deposited, stored and sorted to create a powerful domestic geography, which, in turn sustains a complex and dynamic symbolism and meaning to rooms and spaces.
>
> *(Gurney 2000 p34)*

It is not always clear what is included under the term 'housing', so here I draw, in part, on Ruonavaara's (2018 p179) description as:

> housing choice, homemaking, homelessness, the history and organization of social housing, housing equity release, residential segregation, squatting, self-building, privatization of public rental stock, housing policy, neighbouring, neighbourhood community.

DOI: 10.4324/9781032644868-4

Home is undoubtedly 'a special kind of place' (Easthope 2004) that matters for health and wellbeing, and people have a right to live in appropriate homes and housing. Our physical environments can support or inhibit the ways we live in our worlds, and housing has a material impact on our bodies, emotions and spiritual wellbeing (Smith 2019). The World Health Organisation (2007) stipulates homes must be accessible and usable, large enough to guarantee sufficient space to accommodate people of different ages and allow privacy. Housing standards in countries where they exist, however, offer considerable variations in focus and scope suggesting a widespread lack of commitment and political will to tackling this core public health issue (Capasso and D'Allessandro 2021).

A review of housing spaces in nine European countries, for example, found a variety of room size regulations and some countries, including the United Kingdom, Wales, Germany and Denmark, had no minimum size limit (Appolloni and D'Allesandro 2021). Indeed, in the United Kingdom, landlords must ensure low-cost social housing association homes are safe and free from hazards, in a reasonable state of repair, equipped with 'reasonably modern facilities' and are warm enough (Gov UK 2023). The importance of accessibility, which should allow age-related and other adjustments and sufficient space, do not feature. In the United States, while there are health-related standards for individual areas such as mould, there is no standard that covers how the different factors of the physical housing condition and stability, affordability and community impact health (Swope and Hernández 2019, p2). Marginalised groups face cumulative disadvantages worsened by housing insecurity, cost, condition and location. Swope and Hernandez (2019) frame the need for good quality housing for marginalised groups as a human rights issue and draw on Atuahene's (2016) concept of dignity restoration to underline the importance of correcting past injustices.

People with learning disabilities do not typically access paid employment as I discuss below, and with limited income across their lives are likely to be excluded from the housing market. A Scottish government funded review into the housing opportunities and challenges for people with learning disabilities, for example, found people are more likely to live in social housing (52% compared with 21% of the wider population) and less likely to be homeowners or live in a home their family own (39% compared with 66%) (Ormston et al 2017).

For people with learning disabilities, housing is another aspect of life that is done to them, typically without them. For all the talk of agency, choice and independence, there is little meaningful engagement with or consideration for what this means in practice for people with learning disabilities. While the housing people access will be influenced by the health and social welfare infrastructure of the country they live in, the material, social and political resources of the family, if family are involved, will play a central role in shaping people's lives. UNCRPD Article 19 includes a commitment to ensuring disabled people can choose where they live and with whom, and further, should not be obliged to live in a particular living arrangement; however, this is not happening on any scale for people with learning disabilities.

In Australia, for example, despite the large-scale move from institutions since the 1980s and recognition of the inappropriateness of segregation, deinstitutionalisation has been slow and haphazard (Wiesel and Bigby 2015). Less than a decade ago nearly 4000 people were still living in institutions (Wiesel et al 2015). In Taiwan, around 90% of people with learning disabilities live with their families, while the remainder live in residential settings which are increasing in number as deinstitutionalisation is not a state policy (Chen et al 2022, Chou and Schalock 2007). In a study of 6,778 adults living outside the family home in the United States, less than half of participants exercised choice about where or with whom to live (Stancliffe et al 2011). UK-based evidence suggests people's living situation can remain unchanged for years demonstrating further human rights abuses (Blood et al 2024, Quilgars et al 2024).

Decisions about where people live are often made by professionals or family carers and for people still living in the family home can be delayed to the point at which family carers can no longer care due to ageing. Growing mutual interdependency between the parent and person with learning disabilities can become a further complication (Ryan et al 2024a). Examples of people with learning disabilities as carers have been used to forward claims of citizenship for some (Ward 2011), although this is reminiscent of Kanner's attempt to lift only some people out of the human waste bin. Examples of mutual caring between older family carers and people with learning disabilities in their 40s, 50s or even 60s are a clear indication of the failure of social care support, if the situation has arisen because of a lack of viable alternatives. People in residential care will usually have little choice in who they live with, and people with profound and multiple disabilities are likely to have little or no choice (Vehmas and Mietola 2021) and be relegated to inappropriate or inferior housing (Bigby and Fyffe 2009).

The situation is worsening in some areas. A comparison of data from national social care statistics in England, Scotland and Wales suggests residential home moves to independent living may be stalling across the three countries (Hatton 2017). In Ireland, research about the 'rehoming' of people with learning disabilities who lived in institutions, found some people moved into group homes, some remained in the institution and a third group moved into their own home with support (McConkey et al 2016). The latter group benefitted the most from the move and with reduced costs. There was a tiered effect where people who lived in group homes tended to move into individual homes, while those in congregate settings moved to group homes. The authors flag this irony and caution about the long-term nature of these moves, and how the third group may be denied the opportunity to ever live on their own. This limitation is in part related to austerity measures, the lack of available housing and speed related to the implemented deinstitutionalisation process.

Austerity is often bandied about to provide empty and unsustainable accounts or explanations for poor services, allowing support and services to remain poor. Terms like 'personalisation' and 'person-centred care' are also used to deflect from critical engagement in this area, of forensically exploring *why* people's lives remain poor. Indeed, as a nurse participant in one study commented, different terms are used in social care "without any substance behind them" (Sirotkin 2024 p232). At the same time, the careless or ignorant use of words such as 'rehoming' by researchers, as well as health and social care professionals and providers, contributes to the oppression people experience, as discussed in Chapter 2.

In some countries, including the United Kingdom, the turn to individualised funding is part of a broader emancipatory movement of disabled people (Dickinson 2017). While the intention is to provide people with resources to directly buy support and services, have control over their lives and take risks, in practice there are issues around the amount of allocated funding, availability and appropriateness of support and services for people to purchase, and the continuing impact of wider societal attitudes which can obstruct community engagement. We also know people with learning disabilities are not allowed to take risks despite, as we saw in Chapter 3, the risks people face generated by the conditions under which they are forced to live their lives.

In Australia, people who receive more than eight hours of daily support are eligible to live in group homes in clustered and distributed housing (Skoss et al 2024). Parents of adults with learning disabilities in England often manage direct payments which, while this constitutes a responsibility with substantial emotional and administrative labour and budgeting challenges (Brown et al 2018a), is undertaken because it can allow greater choice and control and subsequently, better support. In our *Spinning Plates* project, we found family carers have to shoulder a disproportionate share of the work which was highlighted within the work and administrative mechanics of the project by the lack of the use of care replacement funding as there was no 'replacement care' to draw on (Runswick-Cole et al in press). The operationalisation of policies like individualised funding can also be obstructed by the lack of involvement of people with learning disabilities in developing the initiative (Bigby and Fyffe 2009), and continuing ignorance about people's lives.

In wider housing literature, the relevant housing conditions that influence health have been divided into four categories: residential instability, affordability, housing quality and neighbourhood. These categories interact with one another and other inequalities, reproducing and reifying health inequalities (Swope and Hernández 2019). In this chapter, I draw on a tweaked version of this categorisation and interrogate the housing conditions and wider community lives of people with learning disabilities. This approach makes visible anomalies in the experiences of people who are sometimes protected from the impact of structural inequalities while being subject to conditions that generate alternative and often invisible or ignored health-related disparities.

Residential instability

Housing instability usually refers to issues around frequent moves, difficulties paying rent and the risk of eviction and homelessness (Burgard et al 2012). While data is variable as some people are not counted in the generation of data or may not have family, the overarching tendency for people with learning disabilities to live in the family home in countries without a residential care model, or with a growing residential care model as in the case of Taiwan, remains substantial. Example figures include: 35% of people with learning disabilities in Scotland (Ormston et al 2017) and over 90% of people in Turkey (Kaya and Wehmeyer 2022).

Living at home with family members could be considered a stable housing environment given reduced issues of cost, potential for frequent moves or eviction and homelessness. Residential stability, whether in the family home or independent supported living, can be problematic, however, if it is the wrong kind of home for the person, living with people they may not want to live with and/or supported by people they may not want to support them. Indeed, Spagnuolo et al (2025) highlight how people with learning disabilities can experience family support as coercive as actions can undermine opportunities for self-determination. Instability is also introduced by the inevitable time limit on how long family carers can support their relative. There is a tendency, as we saw in Chapter 1, to assume if people are clean, well fed and safe, this is good care. This removes aspirations and generates static lives rather than lives which are growing, the definition of a good life (Ryan et al 2024a). Boredom is a strong feature in the lives of people with learning disabilities and this can relate to the organisation of support and housing environments, including living in the family home.

It remains unclear about who is responsible for supporting people with learning disabilities to plan where to live, coordinate support and troubleshoot when things go wrong. Co-production work involving people with learning disabilities, family carers, academics, social care professionals and commissioners in *Growing Older* was dogged by the unanswered questions 'where are the social workers?' and 'who is responsible to support people to plan ahead?' These questions are key given the fragility of care and support arrangements (Ryan et al 2024a).

In the United Kingdom, an enhanced role has developed for community and voluntary sector organisations due to over a decade of austerity-related budget cuts (MacPherson et al 2023). The severest cuts have been in 'the most deprived areas' of social care spending (Hastings et al 2015) and the impact on the wellbeing of people with learning disabilities and family carers has been substantial (Malli et al 2018). We know people are likely to be living on low incomes and in poorer housing than their non-disabled peers, in situations that are characterised by hybridised and precarious arrangements pulled together from left over remnants of support (Power and Bartlett 2018).

There are further anomalies in the evidence. For example, in high-income countries with welfare care systems, neighbourhood deprivation does not impact on the quality of life of people with learning disabilities in the same way it impacts on non-disabled people and may not contribute to health inequalities (Cooper et al 2011). It may be people with learning disabilities are protected from some of the effects of deprivation as an outcome of the control and potentially coercive practices they live under, while experiencing other non-visible effects of constrained, or 'soft' institutionalised lives.

Otherwise 'housed' or homeless

People with learning disabilities are overrepresented among homeless groups and can be even more vulnerable to financial, emotional and sexual abuse within this context. They can, further, find it difficult to move out of homelessness. There is a lack of research in this area, however, and prevalence rates vary. Durbin et al (2018) for example, found between 12% and 39% of homeless people had learning disabilities in nine studies conducted in United Kingdom, Japan, USA and Netherlands, although the authors highlight limitations to the research which include different criteria and measures used to identify people with learning disabilities.

One of the problems homeless people face is service providers may not be equipped to provide appropriate and accessible services because of a lack of awareness about learning disabilities, fragmented systems and a lack of healthcare and housing support (Thurman et al 2023). A Canadian study that involved seven co-researchers with learning disabilities and experience of homelessness found that this group faced significant disadvantages again because of a lack of awareness about learning disabilities and siloed ways of working by relevant stakeholders (Schormans et al 2024). The authors conclude (again) that more joined up working is needed to effectively support this group.

We know people with learning disabilities are overrepresented in prison populations although again figures vary due to differences in definitions and measures, as well as healthcare and justice systems (Hellenbach et al 2017). There are vulnerabilities within criminal justice systems and prison settings due to the lack of accessible information and associated lack of understanding about criminal justice processes. People with learning disabilities are more likely to be apprehended, found guilty and receive longer sentences (Glaser and Deane 1999, Gulati et al 2018). In prison, they are likely to experience victimisation from fellow inmates and have a lower likelihood of being visited by a doctor or family members (Talbot 2010). They are again denied support opportunities available to people without learning disabilities as they are excluded from rehabilitation programmes that aim to reduce recidivism. As we saw in Chapter 3, in relation to family reunification programmes, people are effectively denied the support and opportunities to develop knowledge and understanding to effectively live their lives, offering further evidence of generative epistemic injustice.

There is, further, a clear lack of attention to people with learning disabilities in this area which suggests a lack of interest. In an international review of research published since 2000 about people with learning disabilities and prisons, García-Largo et al (2020) found only 13 papers published internationally. Furthermore, none of the papers mentioned screening for learning disabilities within prison. The authors (García-Largo et al 2020 p8) argue for more comprehensive screening of prisoners and the development of tailored courses for prisoners with learning disabilities, arguing that "prison is a unique opportunity to address the needs of people with ID". The lack of screening again suggests a lack of interest in focusing on the issue of wrongful incarceration, while the exclusion from rehabilitation programmes is another form of structural violence. Indeed, 'habilitation' programmes have been suggested for prisoners with learning disabilities; the persistent lack of support and opportunities means 'rehabilitation' programmes are not appropriate (Glaser and Deane 1999). The suggestion that prisons provide a unique opportunity to address people's needs is puzzling given the failure of the institutionalisation programme to effectively support people with learning disabilities to lead good lives. Perhaps it offers an opportunity to habilitate people, though given the precedence, one that is unlikely to materialise.

There is a question around whether people with learning disabilities should be incarcerated in prisons at all. The intolerance of diversity that underpins people's lives and relationships is ignored, and the impetus is again on people with learning disabilities to reform and become like other people (Glaser and Deane 1999). The criminal justice system is clearly not prepared to consider learning disability and the inherent impact this identity has on the lives of people. In effect, normalisation has "become an ideology of convenience" as it allows people to be incarcerated because they did the crime (Glaser and Deane 1999 p353). It has elsewhere been argued that US prisons have become a de facto ghetto, a new type of institution for people with learning disabilities (Smith 2005).

In addition to formal incarceration, there are also instances where people are held in hospital Section 136 suites because of a lack of appropriate housing in England. For example, 26-year-old Declan Morrison died after spending 10 days in a unit designed for a maximum of 24 hours stay (UK Judiciary 2024a), and another young man, AP was recently awarded substantial damages after spending 340 days in a similar space (Bindmans 2025).

Affordability (and availability)

This category, which I have extended to include availability, generates further contradictions. Social exclusion, discrimination and stigma are experienced across all types of housing, and people with the highest support needs experience an unequal burden of housing disparities (Roebuck 2021). These disparities relate to broader structural inequalities, including the restriction of choices through policies and national or regional government funding frameworks (see, for example, O'Donnell et al 2023). As we saw above, institutionalisation continues in many countries (Roebuck 2021, Walmsley and Jarrett 2019) often due to a lack of alternative housing options (O'Donnell et al 2023).

People with learning disabilities can be excluded from the social housing market in some countries because of the complexity of the application process, a lack of accessible information and housing advice (Quilgars et al 2024). People, families and allies where they exist need accessible and timely information about what options there are and an understanding of rights to ensure people live where they want to live, on their own or with people they want to live with (Bowey and McGlaughlin 2007, Ryan et al 2024a). This is a premise most people take for granted. We know people with learning disabilities in England enjoy renting their own home, in particular "the beauty of privacy, safety, and a general lack of surveillance and intrusion from other people" (Quilgars et al 2024 p367). Given the levels of surveillance people are subject to throughout their lives, being able to shut the front door and experience some privacy fulfils a basic need. The model of independent supported living in the United Kingdom, however, can involve 24-hour support in shared housing with groups of up to six people or more living together. We saw in Chapter 3 how provider rules can include leaving bedroom doors open underlining the surveillance within people's homes. While housing and support within this model are usually provided independently of each other ostensibly to offer more choice, in practice people face limited choices about where to live and moving house can be reactive rather than carefully planned (Blood and Ribenfors 2024, Salmon et al 2019).

For Roebuck (2021), clarity and consistency around the definition of different housing models could help although this risks further 'othering' people with learning disabilities with the weight of more social care-related terms and jargon. Housing is a universal human need, and the WHO definition outlined above is, or should be, comprehensive enough to incorporate the needs of people with learning disabilities.

I noted earlier how people typically have lower incomes in part due to their exclusion from the job market, not being able to undertake paid work, and often higher support needs. This limits access to affordable housing and we know there are gaps in housing options open to people with learning disabilities. Indeed, in Australia, there have been moves towards people with profound disabilities living in larger housing blocks because of a lack of funding for individual support (Bigby and Fyffe 2009). A US review of Federal programs related to housing for people with learning disabilities and/or autistic people found programmes were seriously limited in scope and capacity to provide housing assistance (Paode 2020).

A sense of realism in relation to their home and housing is apparent in research involving people with learning disabilities. One participant in a Canadian study was happy in her flat while recognising there was little option to move given it had taken ten years on a waiting list to move to her current home (O'Donnell et al 2023). Another participant described how an alternative option of housing, the 'roommates programme', which allows for more independent living in privately rented housing was too expensive, so she was looking for an alternative with the expectation "it takes about 10-20 years just to get a one bedroom" (O'Donnell et al 2023 p10). Participants in a UK-based study of people's experiences of renting housing described being encouraged to accept the first or second rental they viewed:

Q: It sounds like there was a lot of pressure to just pick something?
A: Yeah, yeah, just go for this tower block, who cares whether you like it or not, you know…. (Renter 22)

(Quilgars et al 2024 p365)

'Affordability' may not be a direct issue for people in receipt of social care support and people may not be aware of how much rent they pay (Quilgars et al 2024). To consider if a room, flat or a house is affordable involves a set of reflections and decision making that people may not be able to engage with, either through reduced capacity to understand or because of a lack of accessible information and support to negotiate public housing processes. People are kept ignorant of their rights or opportunities that could be open to them, again in a form of generative epistemic injustice. Paode (2020) concludes people are effectively precluded from living and being supported in their own homes and warns the increasing population of older people with learning disabilities in the United States will be at risk of homelessness or (re) institutionalisation.

In Australia, the move to the National Disability Insurance Scheme which aimed to increase the choice and independence of disabled Australian citizens, has led to an estimated unmet need for affordable housing for between 83 and 122,000 people with private rental beyond the reach of most people (Wiesel 2015). This neoliberal policy further generates more pressure on family members, where they exist, who have to navigate the system and advocate for their relatives with learning disabilities. Despite high levels of funding, the National Disability Insurance Scheme has widened inequalities as people in areas of economic disadvantage lack support to effectively access the scheme (Malbon et al 2022). Home sharing and shared equity schemes have been suggested to improve affordability outcomes and improve the use of existing housing stock (Wiesel at al 2015). These strategies can be misused, however, and presented as enhancing social connections rather than the cost-saving exercises they may be.

The disconnect between policy rhetoric and practice in the light of a lack of resources is not unusual; however, there is a peculiar layer of deceit here. For all the talk of autonomy, choice and independence, the extent to which opportunities are so easily removed, of switching from arguments that people can choose where they live to home-sharing schemes with little possibility of moving in the future, is accepted and presented as acceptable. A similar deceit or sleight of hand can be seen in the history of deinstitutionalisation in the Nordic countries in the late 1990s when Denmark removed the term 'institution' from regulations and statistics, and Finland reclassified existing facilities (Tøssebro et al 2012). The lack of available individual homes and the building of group homes can lead to a take it or leave it attitude, and many people take the group home (Tøssebro et al 2012). This removes any consideration of choice as the offer of one option does not constitute a choice.

Housing quality

Reference to housing standards in some countries are welcome although, again with the caveat, these may not be adhered to (Swope and Hernandez 2019). In Ireland, for example, the strategy of the National Housing Strategy for Disabled People (2022–2027) identifies key themes which include accessible, affordable housing, appropriate information, interagency collaboration and raising awareness of disabled people's effective community participation (Gov.IE 2023). Sensible, straightforward and clear statements. An absence of funding to meet these standards (Sheerin et al 2024), and the absence of political will to ensure the appropriate funding is available and conditions enshrined in the UNCRPD are implemented and upheld, however, leaves an acceptance of impoverished conditions of living. There is often little consideration of ageing and the provision of accessible housing for older age (Ormston et al 2017, Ryan et al 2024a). Being able to age in place, for example, should not be determined, as it currently can be by environmental factors and staff training (Northway et al 2017).

People with learning disabilities are more likely to live in areas of deprivation. However, unlike the wider population in these areas, this does not seem to impact on access to healthcare. Instead, it is suggested that the:

> biological, developmental and access problems associated with IDs are so extensive and make such a powerful contribution to the health inequalities that adults with IDs experience, that any impact because of deprivation is trivial by comparison and cannot be detected in a population size of just over 1000.
>
> *(Cooper et al 2011 p319)*

Locating the failings within the person rather than generative epistemic injustices is a damning interpretation of the difficulties people with learning disabilities experience. Cooper et al (2011) offer the possible protective influence of living at home with a family carer who prioritises their wellbeing as an explanation for the discrepancy. Overall, however, they make the point that if living in areas of deprivation does not impact on people with learning disabilities, focusing attention on this area could generate further inequalities for people who do not live in these areas.

The quality of housing, including the aesthetic qualities of place can significantly impact people who, for example, may not be able to open windows to circulate fresh air, turn off bright lights or reduce noise (Smith 2019). The design and occupation of housing has been linked to issues of social justice given how the resulting distress can influence how people are judged and treated (Smith 2019 p154). Creating a home environment that enables participation and control should include consideration of the shape and design of the building, lighting, sound, distribution of spaces, materials, access and engagement with outside spaces. It is not clear how people's sensory needs can be accommodated or are even considered in homes that people share with others, and pets can be prohibited due to tenancy rules (Bould et al 2018).

One ethnographic site in *Growing Older* was an inner-city service in the process of development for ten people with profound and multiple learning disabilities (Ryan et al 2024a). Our research revealed the complexities around the design and development of this service and the gap in current research and practice literature regarding best practice guidelines for commissioning and designing housing for older people with learning disabilities with complex health needs. A key tension was around trying to create 'homeliness' in an environment that needed to engage with and support the physical health, emotional and sensory needs of people living there. The position of a 'nurses station' was a focus of tension as this was felt to medicalise what was someone's home. The impact of the quality of the space, and the impact of that quality on the people who live there is key.

It is clear some people will never 'feel at home' where they are currently living (Smith 2019). People are denied the opportunity to have space, quiet and freedom in their homes. Indeed, there can be barriers to making homes homely, particularly in the shared spaces outside of individual bedrooms, such as the living room, kitchen or even corridors (Chinn et al 2024). Even if people could choose how their bedroom was decorated, there could be unresolved issues that caused the person distress. For example, Belinda was bothered by a crack across her bedroom wall:

When: This happened a while ago.
Where: In my bedroom.
Who: No one did it, it just stays there. Just a crack, you get used to it.
What: My room changed. Is it getting fixed? It is upsetting.
Why: Why am I waiting for it to be fixed? It is taking a while to fix it. It is frustrating. I want this to change.

(Chinn et al 2024 p9)

Homes were also disrupted by staff spaces, rotas and notices, and sections designated out of bounds. The authors conclude that people had to put up with where they were and make the best of it as something worse could always be around the corner (Chinn et al 2024 p11).

It is possible for people with learning disabilities to live on their own with support and create a homely home as we found in *Growing Older*:

> "You've got a lovely home, Z", I say. "I do, don't I", says Z proudly. I think that's what "house-proud" looks like. The place feels homely, simple, but warm (figuratively and literally as the heating is on) and lived in … "Z is very proud of it [the house]", says B, "yeah, I hope I can stay here forever and ever", says Z. (ISL_2, ethnography notes 26 October 2021)
>
> *(Ryan et al 2024a p31)*

However, some participants lived in stable and affordable housing where they were dissatisfied, sometimes for years and with no apparent action to facilitate their move at the time of the research. Some participants lived with people they did not like, or in environments which were ill-suited to them. One participant recently moved home as she wanted to live somewhere quieter.

> When I get to [participant's] room I ask if I should close the door and she [participant] says "yeah, close it". With the door closed, the room feels much cosier and calmer. The door is a two-part situation, with stops at the bottom on both sides. I doubt C can close and open it herself ... The house is noisy ... I then remember C moved to this house recently, so I ask her about that ... "Remind me why you wanted to leave the last place?" "It was because of M, he was always making noises, was loud. Was getting on my nerves" C says. "And is it better here?" I ask. "Not really" C says. (ISL_1, Ethnography notes 7.6.2022)
>
> *(Ryan et al 2024a p34)*

Smith (2018) in her research with people with acquired brain injury considers the 'home' environments of this group offering further analytic insight into the importance of the material and aesthetic quality of these spaces. She describes how the "visual cues of home are juxtaposed with other visual cues indicating alternative ways of life to mainstream society" (Smith 2019 p153). What is key is the atmosphere and the space which allow feelings of connectedness, warmth, comfort, relaxation and freedom that many people can take for granted.

The recognition of these fundamental aspects of home and the disregard for them in relation to people with learning disabilities is a further form of violence. For example, Belinda was not allowed a door key to her own home and had to knock on the back door for staff to let her in (Chinn et al 2024).

The move towards personalisation in high-income countries has been criticised for promoting consumption-focused individualisation at the expense of relational and collective forms of support and care (Power et al 2022). Dominant models of housing and support shape the living conditions for people with learning disabilities which of course dispels any myth that people can choose where they live. People were not involved in decisions around deinstitutionalisation and little attention has been paid to their views about where and how they would like to live. People have, instead, become monetized:

> Individuals therefore began to carry a monetary "value" for local authorities, both a sum of capital to invest in new housing and facilities, and a revenue grant to cover the costs of their care and support. The relationship between an individual and the financial investment they attracted from the state had never been so evident. The money attached to an individual became known in local authority and NHS jargon as their "dowry".
>
> *(Jarrett 2022 p125)*

Costs have an impact on decision making around where and with whom people live, as economies of scale in terms of people living together. A lack of understanding and clarity remains around the size of homes people would like to live in, or would thrive living in. This is, in part, because local authorities, commissioners, providers or family members dominate the decision-making space, and limited research addresses this question with people with learning disabilities. We saw earlier how people were fatalistic about their chances of finding somewhere they wanted to live or absorbed current unhappiness because what lay ahead could be worse.

Decision makers are influenced by costs, safety and lean into an uncritical preference for soft institutionalisation. House sharing across the life course with strangers is expected and unchallenged practice for people with learning disabilities. Some countries introduced prescriptions around the maximum number of people with learning disabilities who should house-share, or the number of individual apartments in a building (Tøssebro et al 2012). In Sweden, for example, in the 1990s, clustered individual apartments were developed with living room, bedroom, kitchen and bathroom, located on residential streets with no more than three to five apartments per building. While people became more visible in their neighbourhoods, this was not accompanied by the anticipated increase in community participation and belonging, leading to Tøssebro (2016 p116) describing "the revolution that disappeared". The shift from national to local government funding in both Sweden and Norway led to fiscal strain and cancelled funding, and there has been a creep back towards larger groups of people living together, although more so in Norway where there are not clear government guidelines and groups of up to 25 people living together have been reported (Tøssebro et al 2012). In Sweden, group homes can still have an institutional feel to them (Svanelöv and Talman 2021).

Steps towards creating the conditions for people to lead good lives are rolled back as accommodation size is driven by neoliberalism and social care cuts, often presented as beneficial for people with learning disabilities (Kittelsaa and Tøssebro 2011). The pattern in Norway is mirrored in Finland and Denmark where large group homes or cluster facilities with an institutional feel are being introduced under the guise of it being easier to provide professional support (Tøssebro et al 2012). While the ideology of community care continues in Nordic countries, in practice there are conflicting trends (Tøssebro et al 2012). Evidence from a number of countries point to what are effectively warehousing practices around the 'placement' of people with learning disabilities in homes that are a better fit with the resources rather than genuine attempts to ensure movement towards people having control and autonomy over where they live (Bigby and Fyffe 2009, Vehmas and Mietola 2021).

A review of older people with learning disabilities in Ireland suggests congregate settings may be more amenable to age-related modification with monies again pooled to overcome the lack of resources (Sheerin et al 2024). This 'doubling up' is a common strategy among marginalised groups more widely in the United States where the cost benefits can lead to overcrowding and associated adverse health outcomes (Swope and Hernandez 2019). Small-staffed homes can provide a better environment for people ascribed as having severe or profound learning disabilities although the importance of basic material and social resources as well as experienced staff is necessary (Mansell and Beasley 1993). Care homes remain part of the housing mix for people with learning disabilities, particularly for older people, again with cost being a factor as people currently living independently can be offered less costly care home places (Stevens 2004).

Where people want to live and with who are not easy to answer questions, not least because people are often not asked in ways they can answer, or supported to answer in ways they can, and because of distorted scholarship in this area. One Australian study found people wanted to live near their peers in large groups in the community (Shaw et al 2011). A shift to what has been described as a core and cluster model has been identified in Scotland, with positive reports that it encourages independence and community participation (Ormston et al 2017). Six participants in a Canadian study said they would like to live in apartments, and of these, five wanted communal spaces with other people to build social ties. Other factors included good public transport, close to green spaces and shops and opportunities to join in activities in the local community.

The cluster living model has been criticised by academics because of lower support levels, greater staffing inconsistency, less access to activities and greater restrictive management practices (Emerson 2004, Mansell and Beadle-Brown 2009). A wider concern is that these more congregate models represent a return towards institutional practices (Ormston et al 2017) and there are higher premature death rates in congregate settings as we saw in Chapter 2. The mark of disposability runs deep in settings that lack love, understanding and recognition.

The normative housing model in the Global North is based on autonomous people, work, relationships, families and community engagement. Given these activities remain largely unattainable for people with learning disabilities, it is concerning people can be denied opportunities to live with others in spaces that while unconventional, may offer freedom, opportunities, safety and security. The question of size is also complicated by confusion between historic memories of institutionalisation, the dominance of certain approaches or voices in disability research which do not include people with learning disabilities, and contradictions and tensions around the availability of funding, resources and housing. We concluded in *Growing Older* that there is no best type of home or living arrangement for people with learning disabilities. It is important people live where they want to live, on their own or with people they want to live with, supported by people they like and who like them, and have lives that are growing.

Fully staffed group homes can have better outcomes in management and some health indicators although independent living or small group living has better outcomes for cost, choice and community activities (Felce et al 2008). Furthermore, the quality of congregated living can vary greatly. In Turkey, for example, the alternative to living with family is group homes or 'care and rehabilitation centres' which tend to be multi-storey buildings with three people per room (Kaya and Wehmeyer 2022).

An established model of support in the United Kingdom, Shared Lives, is where people with learning disabilities (and other marginalised people such as care leavers or people with mental ill health) live with another family in their homes or spend breaks with Shared Lives carers. Around a third of these schemes are run by local authorities and the rest by private providers. This model aims to support people to lead good lives and Shared Lives carers are supposed to be carefully matched to the person with learning disabilities and support the person to become part of their local community (Brookes et al 2024, Callaghan et al 2017). There are similar schemes in the USA, Canada and Europe (Brookes et al 2024). Two Shared Lives schemes in different parts of the country formed part of the ethnographic study in *Growing Older*. While some people were thriving as part of an alternative family, Shared Lives carers will, of course, grow older generating familiar issues around future planning. We also found, in one area, day centre attendance was part of the 'care package'. Instead of living an ordinary life with another family, the person attended a day centre for three or four days a week. This day centre comprised of one room in a large building with a television on in the corner all day. People of all ages attended, and some people were clearly bored. There were few appropriate activities for older people. This is another example of duplicity, as the segregated and largely poor day centre setting contradicts the apparently mainstream Shared Lives approach and values. One commissioner of services who took part in the project said:

> And I keep thinking and going back to that Adult Family Placement – those days when it was Adult Family Placement – because I think things changed from then when it moved to Shared Lives. And there's a focus around having to have the day provision element. I think it loses that sense of being part of the family, when you start looking at the fact that somebody needs to have a day provision or respite. (SL_1)
>
> *(Ryan et al 2024a p33)*

Shared Lives schemes are attractive to local authorities because they offer value for money and are presented as a positive form of post-institutional life, despite the inappropriate fit with the much-worn phrases of autonomy, choice and control. Just as people are not generally expected to house-share across their lifetimes, they are also not expected to live with another family. While the approach clearly works in some instances, the broad-brush presentation of it as a laudable alternative way of living needs more critical scrutiny.

Neighbourhood, home and belonging

Neighbourhood is an important component of housing. A neighbourhood, with parks and open spaces, good transport links and a strong sense of social connectedness can generate a trusting environment, widening people's lives in terms of physical, social, emotional and epistemic access (Capasso and D' Alessandro 2021, Swope and Fernandez 2019). For people with learning disabilities who are likely to experience enduring social, cultural and personal discrimination, a trusting environment is key. However, support offered by neighbours and within neighbourhoods can be variable, ranging from close ties and practical assistance to abuse and bullying (Chinn et al 2024, Power and Bartlett 2018). Indeed, we need to unpack the assumptions that overlay the notion of community living and be careful about making judgements about the possible 'tenderness and care' non-disabled neighbours may exhibit which could be interpreted as disrespectful or a demonstration of power differentials (Dijker et al 2011).

Following Hall (2010), I argue it is important to question the focus on 'successful inclusion' for people with learning disabilities without a clear sense of what this looks like. Indeed, in the United Kingdom, independent supported living, perceived to be a marker of successful inclusion, can lead to people becoming more socially isolated than when they lived with family or in an institutional setting because of a lack of regular contact with people (Jackson 2011).

Belonging is a basic human need (Nind and Strnadová 2020). Meaningful community interactions provide people with opportunities to develop new skills, taking us back to the importance of a life that is growing. When talking about their community life, five participants with learning disabilities in an Australian study described moments marking periods of growth rather than the attributes of the place (le Goullon 2022). Drawing on John Dewey's work on community, time, associations and shared aesthetic experiences were identified as central to belonging. These experiences are apparent in this extract from *Growing Older* about C's pride and apparent contentedness in showing the researcher around their neighbourhood.

> It is a beautiful, warm, sunny day and the town where C lives is lovely, so we (researcher and participant) are going to go for a stroll and have coffee out. As I approach the flats where C live, I can see him and T [support worker] waiting

> at the gate … "Hello!" "Hello! Hi, C, hi, T!" … Then T says "right, C is all set, he has some money to treat you to a coffee. He knows where he wants to go ... There is a café in a garden centre, C likes it there". (ISL_2, ethnography notes 23 March 2022)
>
> *(Ryan et al 2024a p33)*

Participation in community life has been divided into category, structure and level of participation; whether the activity is employment or political activity, segregated or mainstream, brief, an encounter or participation (Simplican et al 2015). Few examples of convivial or fleeting encounters have been found in relation to people with learning disabilities and when they happen, can be repeat encounters where people have developed some familiarity (Weisel and Bigby 2016).

Participating in community activities may not lead to a sense of belonging which involves connections between people, places, objects, animals, practices and ideas (Weisel and Bigby 2016) and is messy and shifting. Belonging, or a feeling of being in place (Mee and Wright 2009), involves collectivity and mattering. Participants with learning disabilities in *Flourishing Lives* challenged the idea that they were simply recipients of support, describing how they gave back to others by volunteering, fundraising, supporting others, being kind, cheerful and loving (Ryan and O'Brien 2024).

Hall (2010) outlines examples of learning disability 'exclusive' places which are safe and creative spaces for people to come together in a shared endeavour (a theatre group and arts and crafts organisation). Companionship, support, a calm environment and being productive are important features of these spaces:

> To belong is to feel attached, to feel valued, and to have a sense of insiderness and proximity to "majority" people, activities, networks and spaces. And it is arguably only with people with IDs (with support and advocacy) taking part in continuous active processes of insiderness and proximity, perhaps through projects such as those outlined above, that the deeply-set structures of society can be gradually dismantled.
>
> *(Hall 2010 p56)*

There is a conundrum here, that again is difficult to disentangle because of the stronghold of social care speak, jargon and exclusionary language. I earlier discussed a flaw in the Shared Lives model which involved day centre provision undermining the ordinary life ethos of the approach. However, spending time with similar others can be a space of bounded safety for many people, the comfort of feeling accepted, of understanding language use, jokes, of recognising shared experiences, of belonging. For people with learning disabilities, certainly in countries like England, there has been a push to fragment communities of people with the process of deinstitutionalisation and subsequently the closing down of day centre provision (Power and Bartlett 2018). The lives of people with learning disabilities are dictated by the latest or dated policy prescriptions and whim of local authorities, commissioners, families and other stakeholders in this space. Those directly impacted are sidelined in these decisions, particularly people with profound and multiple disabilities.

There are myriad examples of belonging in different ways and for different reasons. In *Growing Older* (Ryan et al 2024a), one participant, Geoff, lived with a Shared Lives family in South England and developed a smallholding with various livestock. From a farming background and with a strong love of the outdoors and animals, Geoff, who is in his 70s, works with and manages the smallholding. He is also clearly part of the family he lives with:

> GI's [Shared Lives carer's] parents shoot game. When Gl's parents visit, her dad is really coming to see Geoff and will head down to see him in the fields before seeing anyone else. They have a lot in common and are quite alike in their personalities as well. Geoff will mention him often and will pick up little gifts for him such as a mug with a pheasant on when they were recently in a shop. (SL_2, Ethnography notes 3.11.2021)
>
> *(Ryan et al 2024a p46)*

Belonging necessarily involves a sense of permanency, of home-making practices in the moment and foreseeable future, with conditions such as outside space or pet ownership attached (Mee and Wright 2009, Ryan et al 2024a). It involves accommodation and encouragement, listening to and acting on what is important to people. As we saw in the examples above and in Brison's description of her relationship with Sesha, it also involves reciprocity, kindness and love. There are ways of creating forms of belonging that escape exclusionary politics; where "we find a belonging created through active, hybrid, fragile, and always contested processes that refuse containment" (Mee and Wright 2009 p776).

In the final section of this chapter, I provide a brief excursion into what we know about employment and people with learning disabilities. In writing this book, it did not feel appropriate to include a chapter on employment as I originally planned. The numbers of people in paid work are derisory and, following Chapter 3, it seems counter-intuitive to write yet another chapter about what people with learning disabilities are obstructed from doing. Instead, I provide an overview of key areas relating to employment and draw out some points that add further depth or understanding to issues raised so far across the book.

Employment

Employment matters and is 'intricately linked' with health and well-being (Melzter et al 2020). Indeed, a direct link is made in Article 23 of the Universal Declaration of Human Rights between work and dignity. Evidence suggests there are similar associations between better health and employment for people with learning disabilities as non-disabled people (Eggleton et al 1999, Robertson et al 2019a). We have established that people with learning disabilities are people in the areas of health, love, intimacy and employment. In the area of employment is also the now-familiar caveat of research inconsistencies around definitions and what constitutes employment.

Employment offers better health outcomes, financial cost-benefit issues and should support an equality agenda. Well-established benefits of working include earning money, having a sense of purpose, structure, developing relationships and a better quality of life (Almalky 2020). For David, the importance of work lies in "getting paid for it. [Laughs] Keeping fit. Learning" (Merrells et al 2019 p16), while a participant in Timmons et al (2011 p293) study described how:

> I felt like a "somebody" working in higher enterprise and going to work and then coming back. I felt like a person, like someone normal would feel like in a job and everything. And I'm helping the community, helping people with their groceries. I felt good about that.

The number of people with learning disabilities in paid employment, however, remains resolutely low. In England, the paid employment rate of people with learning disabilities has fallen to an all-time low of 4.7% (Hatton 2024).

Low employment rates can be due to discriminatory attitudes on the part of employers, people can lack confidence with low aspirations set from childhood, little or no careers advice, work experience or vocational training while at school. Young people can feel excluded from decision making about their future and unable to access meaningful opportunities beyond volunteering (Mogensen et al 2024).

At the same time, there is a tendency to over-idealise paid employment and a lack of recognition for other contributions people make. Melbøe and Hardonk (2022) argue presenting paid employment as a key criterion for citizenship renders voluntary work invisible. However, linking employment (paid or voluntary) to notions of citizenship again brings us back to the slippery slope to Kanner's human waste bin. Elevating some people based on 'productivity' further pushes down on those unable to undertake any form of employment. Volunteering can, however, be acknowledged in terms of providing a sense of belonging, developing competence, relationships and contributing, and may happen alongside paid or sheltered employment (Melbøe and Hardonk 2022).

From employers' perspectives, considerations around employing people with learning disabilities include safety, attendance, the availability of support services, 'behavioural problems' and punctuality (Ellenkamp et al 2016). Different people, circumstances and experiences have been identified as important at points along the journey to employment and include: family members and schools raising work expectations and confidence; job developers facilitating job hunting, matching and supporting people in the role; and personal reasons for the person around earning money, feeling a sense of achievement and the quality of social relationships (Timmons et al 2011).

Some countries have legislation to promote inclusion in the workplace. In Canada, for example, federally regulated industries are mandated and there is an emphasis on employment-support organisations, although family members and social networks can be a key feature in gaining and sustaining employment (Petner-Arrey et al 2016). Nordic labour policies are based on the premise that all members of society should have equal opportunities and support, and yet the employment situation of people with learning disabilities remains poor (Gjertsen et al 2021). In Iceland, segregated workplaces have remained unchanged for decades and it has been commented that the only way to leave such a setting is through death. The emphasis in Iceland, Norway and Sweden is on strengthening the person rather than addressing barriers in the workplace (Gjertsen et al 2021). This is in line with research recommendations in other areas and is antithetical to the widely adopted social model of disability which links oppression to external structures and processes. It appears whichever area under consideration and from whatever perspective the problem lies with people with learning disabilities.

Hermeneutical injustice is apparent in relation to the introduction in the Swedish welfare system provision under the *Act concerning the Support and Service for Persons with Certain Functional Impairments* (1994). The provision includes access to daily work which is compensated for by an allowance often equivalent to a cup of coffee. This provision acts to oppress and constrain, however, as one study found participants are left without epistemic resources to understand the meaning of their working lives. Participants described worrying about the financial impact on their lives if they lost their jobs (Kalman et al 2016). Interventions that aim to increase the participation of disabled people in the workforce can be interpreted as corrections in the structure of capital (Mészáros 2008) rather than meaningful change. Working for a day for a cup of coffee is exploitative and people are obstructed from understanding this, underlining their social powerlessness.

Other forms of support include parents who offer advice, encouragement, drawing on their social networks to find jobs and then work as job coaches supporting employment. This labour can be draining, however, and family carers can end up worn out (Pettner-Arry et al 2016). Schools can play a key role in encouraging and supporting employment aspirations (Garrels and Sigstad 2021), particularly through work placements and careers advice, though this is often classroom-based (Timmons et al 2011). A focus on the importance of motivation levels in succeeding to gain and maintain employment has been highlighted, leading to a conclusion that motivational strategies may be important to develop in supported employment support agencies (Rose et al 2005). Strong motivation helped some people recover from poor work experiences and find alternative employment while others decided to no longer pursue paid work (Timmons et al 2011).

Employment models include sheltered employment which involves training and prevocational services, supported employment and employment in the open labour market. Jahoda et al (2008), for example, discuss how people with learning disabilities need to understand the culture and unwritten workplace rules to sustain employment. This can be demanding for people and seems to be an unnecessary bar to attain. In a particularly gruelling articulation, one employment model, the 'place, train and maintain' approach, involves profiling to identify the work-related goals of the person within the context of their broader life aspirations. Then the person is marketed to an employer and their needs discussed. A key worker conducts an analysis of the job, breaking the task down into component parts and encouraging the person to practice each task until it is mastered (Jahoda et al 2008 p2). Given the consistently low employment rates of people with learning disabilities, it is probably time to acknowledge that this is not an effective model.

Sheltered employment is a euphemism for segregated employment and involves considerably less pay and hours of work. Segregated work settings contravene the UNCRPD and can be exploitative as they can involve unpaid work such as packaging gifts with little anticipation of moving into paid employment (Gjertsen et al 2021). Little movement has been found between working in sheltered settings and competitive, community-based employment (Siperstein et al 2014). Indeed, sheltered employment can be a barrier to gaining work in the open labour market (Nevala et al 2019).

Higher levels of job satisfaction, quality of life and autonomy have been found among people who are competitively employed although there is contradictory evidence around paid employment and the development of wider relationships. Kocman and Weber (2018), for example, found people were more active in their leisure lives than those people in sheltered employment or unemployed groups. Merrells et al (2019) found relationships did not develop, and a US-based study found paid employment helped surface level friendships to develop between colleagues. As one staff member stated:

> … he has some relationships at work. I think work is a strong base for his sort of feeling of belonging and feeling of value. And he has some people there that he has a relationship in that sort of way. I'm not sure he has any strong, really social relationships at work of, "Hey, the weekend's coming up. You want to get together and go do something?" kind of level.
>
> *(Timmons 2011 p293)*

Support in this area also includes employment-support agencies, the quality and competence of whom can be variable. An Australian study focusing on barriers to paid employment involving 51 people with learning disabilities found a lack of holistic support by employment support agencies:

> I used to go through … a job agency. They were not very helpful … they would just say to you "Just look in the paper" or "Do this"—they do not actually properly help you find a job, so it was really hard to find a job for me … .I just reckon they should just sort of maybe help you, not just "Do this and do that, hope you get a job." Just maybe more mental and physical sort of like—help you, make phone calls for you or something. (29-year-old woman, urban, currently working in sheltered employment)
>
> *(Meltzer et al 2020 p93)*

When one participant asked a specialist employment service how she could develop her skills to enable her to go for less menial jobs, she was told this was beyond the remit of the organisation. The constraining of ambition and aspirations is further evidenced by people being diverted into sheltered employment schemes to do work preparation courses including computer training, writing and stocking shelves (Timmons et al 2011). Just one of the four Community Rehabilitation Providers in this study focused on paid employment only with the ethos that people were always job ready and needed support to identify career goals and opportunities.

Potential employers can demonstrate obstructive and discriminatory attitudes and not take job applications from people with learning disabilities seriously. As Grace who works in a patisserie in Australia described:

> And I find it really difficult. Um, because I find it hard to keep up with everything because I know everything has to be done at a certain time … So, um, yeah, so I phoned up, like, last week to see if there's any more shifts, and there haven't been any shifts for me, like, this week,so … yeah.
>
> *(Merrells et al 2019 p16)*

This discouragement could lead to people accepting sheltered employment. Indeed, people enjoy friendships they make in sheltered accommodation, and the confidence developed doing work well, and can 'sabotage' their paid employment opportunities to return to the camaraderie of the sheltered employment programme (Timmons et al 2011). Where people found paid employment, they could feel disrespected and unvalued in the workplace:

> I thought when I first applied for a shop assistant role that I'd be serving customers, that I'd be stocking shelves, doing returns, face up, pricing, on the registers. I thought it was going to be quite varied, but then I mostly would just be stocking shelves.[It was] just cleaning or working in the kitchen, which I did not

> really enjoy, and I wanted to be in more a position where I could feel I'm helping more people … . (30-year-old woman, urban, working in open employment)
> *(Meltzer 2020 p95)*

Support workers can also obstruct people's access to work by not listening or taking their employment seriously. Annika described how:

> And they don't listen to what you're saying to them. That really, really pisses me off [with support] workers – when there's an [issue] and you are trying to tell them what you want and they don't know, they don't listen to you.
> *(Robinson and Idle 2023 p66)*

Participants again described being given entry level jobs with no opportunities for advancement, in roles often subject to economic precariarity. This could lead to considerable disillusionment. A further study of 27 young people in three areas in Australia found participants wanted paid employment, completed various courses and volunteering roles yet were still unable to access work (Mogensen et al 2024). They described being disillusioned with the specialist employment organisations to the extent the research team were asked to help participants:

> Um, so in a job, right, can you teach me how to get a real job? Because I wonder if anyone can help me get a job … I trust my mum, but I'm mainly trusting myself or someone else I know. It's really hard. (Jack
> *(Mogensen et al 2024 p127)*

Another participant described how he wanted to "be more than just a disability person" (Mogensen et al 2024 p127) and several participants discussed how difficult it was to lose the structure of school. The authors conclude there has been minimal change in the experiences of young people leaving school despite decades of research and recommendations, leaving people without meaningful adult lives. The intense boredom that can inhabit lives without structure is illustrated by Anne's description of her day:

> Ah, nothing really. Bored ... [Today] Um, cleaned my house, did my dishes, um, went to the shops, looked around, got some DVDs last night to watch, yeah … get bored so I just go to the shops, but the shops get boring after a while.
> *(Merrells et al 2019 p17)*

Questions are again raised in this area about the quality of published research which can include varying and a lack of definition around measures and measurement, including employment sustainability, a lack of detail about the characteristics of participants, their competence, strengths and educational backgrounds and focus on diagnosis (Nevala et al 2019, Taubner et al 2022). Observational studies about social interactions via the workplace can present descriptions of encounters without any sense of the quality of the engagement (Jahoda et al 2008). There is a tendency for researchers to homogenise the workplace, ignoring the context or recognising supported employees bring their own personal histories and dispositions to work. Indeed, becoming established in the workplace will involve negotiation and likely compromise, and failure at work can be keenly felt, leading to Jahoda et al (2009 p15) suggesting:

> If people themselves can acknowledge the stresses and strains of work, alongside the benefits, then supported employment professionals need to develop a more sophisticated understanding of individuals' socio-emotional needs and strategies for offering appropriate help where it is required.

Concluding thoughts

In the opening paragraph to this chapter, I referred to the powerful domestic geographies of homes, which sustain complex and shifting symbolism and meaning to rooms and spaces (Gurney 2000). The domestic geographies of people with learning disabilities are disrupted, obstructed and subjected to intrusive interventions. People's living space is constricted by provider rules, staff actions and sometimes the actions of housemates. Privacy is trampled through an absence of respect and there are few opportunities or support to move or consider the future.

Employment, which is not essential like housing although matters, is marked by poor employment rates and interventions underpinned by low aspirations and expectations. Sheltered employment programmes, for example, are an early post-institutionalisation relic which are exploitative and segregating. Goodey (2017 p27), when thinking about opportunities for paid employment, highlights the fine line between radical critique and disengagement in the forums where academia and practice meet. There is some irony that academia is beginning to provide employment opportunities for people with learning disabilities. During the *Growing Older* and *Flourishing Lives* projects, we were able to change university processes and procedures to allow paying people for their work and contributions rather than giving shopping vouchers, and Richard Keagan-Bull, a researcher with learning disabilities remains employed at Kingston University (Anderson et al 2023). These projects involved considerable stumbling, the development of new skills, knowledge and understanding for the whole team, the bending of academic conventions and recognition of the importance of adequate funded time and enjoyment. Radical critique can be accompanied by thinking creatively, being bold and doing things differently.

5

FOOD AND EATING

Introduction

In this chapter, food and eating is used as a focus to further reflect upon and expand or develop key arguments and ideas presented in this book. I begin with a consideration of food and eating to see what insights this brings to an unapologetic table. Food consumption is as universal as health, love, relationships and shelter. We all eat and drink. Eating typically involves choices and making decisions, preparing or buying food, cooking and often sharing meals and being together. Shared mealtimes can be a source of pleasure, sociality and belonging, and have been described as dignity-making opportunities for older people (den Uijl et al 2014). Indeed, for Mintz and Du Bois (2002 p102); "next to breathing, eating is perhaps the most essential of all human activities, and one with which much of social life is entwined".

Food insecurity, that is the lack of being able to buy or produce food, is a social determinant of health leading to numerous life-limiting health conditions which include heart disease, hypertension, stroke, chronic obstructive pulmonary disorder and obesity. Food security is defined by the World Bank as "access by all people at all times to enough food for an active, healthy life" (Reutlinger 1986 p1). Food insecurity is an outcome of various factors, including low household incomes and instability in food prices and production (Borras and Mohammed 2020). The global prevalence of undernutrition continues to grow, increasing from 10.6% in 2015 to 10.8% in 2017 while an estimated 40% of the global population is overweight (FAO et al 2019).

There has been a shift to focus on individual households in this area. In 2014, the Rome Declaration on Nutrition asserted "the right of everyone to have access to safe, sufficient and nutritious food, consistent with the right to adequate

DOI: 10.4324/9781032644868-5

food and the fundamental right of everyone to be free from hunger" (FAO and WHO 2014 p1). While class, ethnicity and gender dominate the food-insecure households, disability is also a strong factor although less visible in the more recent consideration of the food sovereignty paradigm which brings critique of capitalism, neoliberalism and dominant Global North nation states to the fore (Borras and Mohammed 2020). In 2002, however, the US Attorney General made improving the nutrition of people with learning disabilities a national priority. One goal of the subsequent and wider call to action to improve the health and wellbeing of disabled people included making people in the United States aware that disabled people can lead long, happy and productive lives. Quite the goal to be setting at the start of the 21st century.

People with learning disabilities are reported to be less likely to eat recommended portions of fruit and vegetables and more likely to have poor diets (Gast et al 2022). A higher prevalence of obesity has been explained by boredom, poor nutrition and over medication (Doherty et al 2020b) and the unlikeliness that people will meet exercise recommendations (Hsei et al 2014, Koritsas and Iocono 2016). Over-medicated and perennially empty lives are not conducive to good health. People with learning disabilities can experience problems swallowing some foods and aspiration-related respiratory illnesses are a key cause of premature death (Redley 2021). Indeed, dietary risks are highlighted as a key, modifiable factor in terms of ameliorating health inequalities and yet despite evidence underlining the effectiveness of interventions that focus on environmental factors, 84% of studies in one systematic review, again, focused on individuals (Dean et al 2021).

Research in this area largely overlooks how mealtimes can be a space of shared enjoyment and sociality. A key theme across this book has been the transformation of the ordinary, the everyday and taken for granted into a confusing and jagged space of social care jargon, contradiction, intervention and abuse, of monstering lives. Food-related research highlights further indignities and disrespect for people with learning disabilities evidenced by the use of language. The term "self-feeders" (Samuels and Chadwick 2006), for example, is used with little reflection, reducing people to either deficit actions and/or disconnection from the wider public of 'self-feeders'. We are, as a research community, complicit in disavowing the ordinary and firmly othering people with learning disabilities.

Support workers again ...

Support staff, who may not necessarily have knowledge of nutritional values and healthy eating, again play a key role when it comes to food and mealtimes. We have repeatedly seen the impact of retention issues, low staff ratios and the poor working conditions experienced by support staff. There are further tensions around choice, autonomy and 'healthy eating'. Who decides *what* someone can eat and when, and how much thought, attention and detail goes into ensuring the person is supported to enjoy food? One support worker at a UK-based day centre commented:

> We give [him] a choice and give him an informed choice … he wants stew and tatties then it's his choice he's an adult. (Paid carer 1)
>
> *(Cartwright et al 2015 p107)*

This contrasts with the refusals we saw in Chapter 3 to support people to express their sexual identities and engage in intimate relationships. Evidence of diet-related poor health is strong, and it may be eating processed food is less work for staff and cheaper than preparing fresh food. People can only choose between available food which may not be nutritional or something they like eating. For example, during the *Flourishing Lives* project, we heard about people being offered the choice of chicken nuggets or chicken dippers for their tea. Support workers may over-compensate in relation to food choices because of the obvious denial of other pleasures. This is borne out by a second participant in the same study stating:

> Food is one of the few oral pleasures that a lot of people with learning disabilities ever get within a mile of. (Project leader 6)
>
> *(Cartwright et al 2015 p110)*

What this support worker meant by this comment is not clear in the published evidence. Few studies focus on the enjoyment of food. Of food as food to be prepared, cooked and shared in different cultural contexts outside the constraints of social care practices and basic sustenance. Research around food consumption can further introduce layers of judgement into the research design as food is often viewed through a healthy eating lens and we fail to see or acknowledge other issues that may emerge during studies.

Eating together or otherwise

Eating together with family and friends is an internationally accepted symbolic activity (Adolfsson et al 2010), which involves being sociable, togetherness, belonging and learning about social and cultural norms. An ethnographic study of the mealtimes of people with learning disabilities who lived in group homes or supported living in Sweden found people appreciated the rare occasions where staff members ate with them:

> According to the staff, food is often a topic of discussion [among the residents], and so were requests to eat together in the common eating area to which those with supported living as well as participants living in the group homes had

access. Tacos were a favourite food. They also began talking about sharing Christmas meals early in the autumn.

(Adolfsson et al 2010 p264)

The authors found people enjoyed talking about food and mealtimes, and there is a refreshing example of someone living in a group home inviting a neighbour in the same home for a meal and then sharing the meal 'in silence'. Restrictions on opportunities for people to share meals were imposed by staff when certain people were seen as unruly or too noisy to eat with others. Wider municipal rules around staff eating food paid for by public funds allocated to people with learning disabilities reduced the opportunities for people to sit down and eat together. This generated feelings of awkwardness on the part of staff who would sit and read a newspaper or do some other distracting activity to not stare at the person eating. Adolfsson et al (2010) found some staff rejected eating with the people they supported or even using the same plates and cutlery. They state the reason for this was not clear. The study found people with learning disabilities wanted more opportunities to eat with other people although this was not always possible outside group homes. In *Flourishing Lives*, we found some parents paid for staff to eat in cafes so their relative was not eating or drinking alone although this was acknowledged as costly and sometimes prohibitive (Ryan and O'Brien 2024). The model of personal assistance or support work drawn up in the wider disabled community does not translate easily to the lives of people with learning disabilities for whom support staff can be a key relationship beyond the support tasks undertaken.

Food and risk

Mealtimes and eating can involve risk for people. Aside from difficulties eating or drinking leading to nutritional and dehydration issues, people can be at risk of choking, asphyxiation or respiratory disease (Ball et al 2012). Strategies to ameliorate these risks include staff support and observation of mealtimes, modifying food and drink to different consistencies, using specialist utensils or interventions such as a percutaneous endoscopic gastrostomy (PEG) feeding tube, and speech and language support. Research suggests nutritional disparities and nutritional behaviour issues may be avoidable among people with learning disabilities (Öztürk and Yabansi Ayhan 2024).

The most common support needs around mealtimes are modified food and "prompting pace and encouragement" (Ball et al 2012 p388). While the former is well-documented and covered by clinical guidelines, the latter is harder for support staff to adhere to (Chadwick et al 2003). Staff are responsible for ensuring food is digestible, of the appropriate consistency, swallowed effectively while enabling people to choose what they want to eat. One study, for example, found a commitment to letting people eat what they want despite possible health risks

(Redley 2021). A support worker participant described how she supported someone who enjoyed toast. This was raised as a choking risk with the Speech and Language therapist, and the advice was to 'try and avoid' foods like toast. The support worker worked around this by cutting the toast into small pieces demonstrating freedom to exercise creativity and flexibility in terms of supporting people to eat and balancing their choice and autonomy against potential health risks. There are complex ways of operationalising choice while ensuring safe and adequate nutrition. This is not feasible, however, when support workers are new or agency staff which, as we have seen, is common practice in a precarious and underfunded social care arena. Examples of risky practices by support workers are evident. For example:

> Shift leader asked if thickener had been stirred into the drink. Agency worker stated No she wasn't aware he had thickener. (N20)
>
> *(Guthrie et al 2015 p128)*

A participant in a Tawainese study of support workers in institutions recounted how:

> … he trembled when I approached him because he didn't trust me. In order to feed him, I spent a lot of time getting to know him so he felt comfortable with me. Unfortunately, he moved to another institution … the new place didn't allow him to eat in his own time and way. He refused or couldn't eat in their way. They used nasogastric intubation and not long later he passed away … .
>
> *(Chen et al 2022 p6)*

Choking is a major cause of death among people with learning disabilities, a risk increased by multiple medication use and antipsychotic drugs. People are three times more likely to have a choking history if they live in community or residential homes which suggests less careful engagement by staff at mealtimes (Manduchi et al 2021). This clearly links to the higher mortality rates we have seen in congregate settings. Support workers' attention is essential in ensuring safe eating and effectively reporting risks; however, staff may not know how to respond to an incident of choking (Manduchi et al 2021).

The reporting of incidents in this area is unsurprisingly inadequate. In a study prompted by a series of deaths through choking in one NHS hospital, incident reports were compared from National Reporting and Learning System (NRLS) data and local data (Guthrie et al 2015). There was little guidance on the rating system for reporting incidents. One local death was marked as 'catastrophic' which juxtapositions the daily grind of often poor care with the peculiar and bureaucratic marking of social murder. It reads as if a staff member has suddenly woken from slumber to note a life has been taken. This takes us back to the reflections by Capri et al (2018) about the Esidemenis Life scandal and the binary appreciation of the lives of people with learning disabilities where the only meaningful statistic is alive or dead.

The reports logged choking incidents as 'personal accident' rather than 'clinical incident' which is inaccurate given medical precedents to choking instances. The NRLS reporting does not request detail about these instances although local reports were prompted to provide more detail. Entries included (with a sadness warning) (Guthrie et al p125):

> client was panicking [sic] struggling to cough or breathe. client had tilted their head back, with their mouth wide open. L28

> He crammed food into his mouth and did not chew suffic [sic]. Appeared unable to breathe, red faced, nose running, tears. L18

> Whilst eating tea the client began to choke and gasp for air. grabbing hold of his throat. He then jumped to his feet and started pointing at his throat his face going red in colour. L5

It is hard to imagine the horror of experiencing these often-repeated incidents and there seems to be little or no consideration of the emotional impact of these events for people with learning disabilities. Guthrie et al (2015) discuss how the reporting system does not allow space for recording the emotional or traumatic impact of these incidents, or the longer-term impacts. This extraordinary positioning of no injury other than death speaks to the erasure of any consideration of trauma in the recording of incidents and the system that underpins it. How people feel and the impact of the incident on them and their relationships with others is ignored, as they are dehumanised. Evidence highlights how people with learning disabilities alerted staff to choking incidents suggesting, again often overlooked, care and attention among and between people being supported.

Guthrie et al (2015 p130) conclude more staff training is necessary alongside 'service user involvement' in the reporting of choking incidents, and more research into influencing factors "to improve treatment and care for service users and develop strategies to mitigate risk". Once again, repeated recommendations for more training and further research which lead nowhere. This begs the question what the point of this research is? As Emerson (2021) states, existing knowledge is sufficient to drive changes in policy and practice, other than the need for more research in the Global South and among ethnic minority populations and people with mild learning disabilities. We know enough to implement what can be small changes to considerably improve the life experiences of people with learning disabilities.

The death of 49-year-old Craig Spiby after choking on a sandwich led to the UK coroner issuing a prevention of future death report that highlighted how Craig's care plan stated he needed to be monitored at mealtimes. However, staff did not have a shared understanding of what 'monitored' meant. There were no clear definitions in the paperwork and staff assumed Craig had fallen asleep, thereby demonstrating no professional curiosity. Staff had no confidence in the emergency first-aid training and there was no training to guard against confirmation bias with people who had a high risk of choking but no previously recorded records of such events (UK Judiciary 2024). Operationalising the term 'monitoring' in the support and care of people with learning disabilities is not a difficult task and there must be myriad support workers and family carers doing just this across the United Kingdom and wider. The lack of this operationalisation, and the numerous deaths that are an outcome of the absence of paying attention, demonstrating curiosity and care, and changing practice after preventable deaths, again constitute social murder.

Related to choking is the likelihood that people with learning disabilities will have none, or fewer, natural teeth than non-disabled people (Anders and Davis 2010, Kinnear et al 2019). A tendency to extract rather than fill teeth offers further evidence of systemic violence. Edentulous, the term for no natural teeth, among people with learning disabilities has been accounted for by the overuse of psychotic medication which can leave mouths dry and susceptible to decay, poor dental hygiene and resistance to dental treatment (Kinnear et al 2019). In some countries, such as Korea, the cost of dental treatment can be difficult to prioritise over other healthcare issues (Lee and Chang 2021). As Kinnear et al (2019), drawing on Hennequin et al (2000) report, people receive more radical dental treatment planning when pharmacological interventions are needed to reduce the chance of the procedure happening again. This study also found no correlation between neighbourhood deprivation and teeth loss. Teeth removal is a preventable inequality which has substantial impact on the quality of life, including the enjoyment of eating, yet this is rarely considered. Neither, it seems, is the use of dentures or dental implants.

I remember reading with horror about the dental experiment that involved giving Swedish children with learning disabilities, who lived in the Vipeholm institution in the 1950s, toffees over a period of nine years to study the effect on tooth decay. A largely unrepentant plaque collector from the study wrote his reflections about the experiment 50 years later. He attributed the high number of citations the study has to the design and execution of the research; the institution enabled well-controlled conditions, and the results were supported by supplementary studies (Krasse 2001).

In responding to criticisms about the ethical implications of the study, he concluded with two trite sayings: the end justifies the means, and it is easy to be wise after the event. While this is not the only example of the abuse of people with learning disabilities or other marginalised people in pursuit of scientific knowledge, there is some poignancy that the unnecessary loss of teeth continues to be replicated 70 years later. Once again, evidence generated from the harm of children and adults with learning disabilities is used to further the health and wellbeing of the mainstream population without benefiting those who were harmed. It is also of note that the children at Vipeholm experienced higher mortality rates during World War Two because of the higher support needs the children had around eating and staff shortages (Seeman 2006). Again, it is not difficult to identify examples of social murder.

Getting the job done

The intimacy and intensity of supported meals for people with profound learning disabilities is substantial as people cannot get away. As Martinsen et al (2008, p537) state "You are locked in. You are not free of it until the meal is over". Mealtimes can become task-based activities with a focus on getting the job done rather than considering the enjoyment of eating and shared mealtimes. Nicholson (2023), through a conversation analysis of recorded mealtimes, found people with profound learning disabilities could show if they were ready to eat:

> Readiness was demonstrated in a number of ways, including eye gaze towards food and/or the staff member, opening the mouth, and reaching for feeding equipment. More generally, stopping other activities and a lack of behaviours demonstrating unreadiness could also signal readiness.
>
> *(Nicholson 2023 p2748)*

Coercion was identified when staff did not wait for a demonstration of readiness before feeding, despite the lowered risks associated with eating when staff wait for readiness cues. Mundane acts of self-determination on the part of the person were obstructed by staff ignoring their actions. The analysis demonstrated how opportunities to talk during mealtimes were also limited by staff taking the opportunity of an open mouth to feed people. The indignity and powerlessness captured here, and endured over time, are almost beyond comprehension.

Surveillance and scrutiny discussed in Chapter 3 is also evident in relation to when, what and where people with learning disabilities eat. An example of this is apparent from the fieldnotes from one study:

> During another morning break I shared a packet of cookies I had purchased with a second young woman. Although we had been sitting apart from anyone else in the canteen, the fact that Louise had accepted and eaten the cookies had been noted by staff and was commented on to me later in the morning. I was told that Louise's parents were concerned about her refusing food of late.
>
> *(Aull Davies 2007 np)*

Cartwright et al (2015) generated interesting considerations around the different spaces people with learning disabilities spend time in and issues of blame that bounce between support workers and family members. Considerations that involved layers of judgement and pejorative statements. For example,

> Some parents will specify to take their kids to soft play and then McDonalds for their tea. (Paid carer 6)
>
> I would say going by the photos that we saw last week on her phone it is not as healthy as it could be at home. (Paid carer 8)
>
> *(Cartwright et al 2015 p111)*

An ethnographic study of mealtimes at day centres based in the United Kingdom found considerable control over the food participants with learning disabilities had access to. In one day centre, people were only offered tea in plastic cups while staff had a choice of tea or coffee in china cups (Aull Davies 2007). Children's food (pies, sausages, beans and chips) and children's treats (sweets, soft drinks and chocolates) were highlighted as favoured to buy. Decorated birthday cakes and family parties instead of restaurant dinners were highlighted as childish, suggesting a pejorative lens as many people may choose food stuffs and treats that could be classed as 'childish'. This is illustrated by one extract in which the participant describes cutting down on chips and liking beans, sausage, scrambled egg, tomatoes. This is interpreted by the author as reflecting a food consumption pattern associated in British culture with children. The term 'pocket money' was further used in this analysis without consideration of the relationship people with learning disabilities have with money or reflection about the micro violence the researcher is inflicting through their words:

> Thus, in general, food preferences tend to weaken the adult social identity of people with learning disabilities. Such ambiguity is compounded by their reported use of pocket money; nearly all said they spent their pocket money on soda pop, sweets and chocolates.
>
> *(Aull Davies 2007 np)*

A question of interventions

Intervention research flourishes around food and eating. It is as if the research community has lifted normative and judgement-laden considerations around nutrition and exercise and applied them to people with learning disabilities in a smorgasbord of studies that lack robustness with few valid and reliable measurements used (Casey and Rasmussen 2013). Let's take a brief foray into this evidence ...

There is an argument that mutual engagement in health-promoting activities can provide a sense of connectedness for people with learning disabilities (Hatzikiriakidis et al 2024). Learning to cook and appreciate food has been highlighted as a way of encouraging healthy eating, although, again, judgements creep in as Aull Davies (2007) reports lessons can focus on less healthy options such as fish fingers, baked beans and other tinned foods. In Sweden, an intervention that focused on increasing the knowledge of people with learning disabilities and support workers around healthy eating and exercise, found parts of the intervention were positive. For example, group meals could create feelings of belonging and staff described some benefits from the knowledge they gained about exercise and healthy eating (Umb Carlsson 2021). There were, however, obstacles and clunkiness to the approach; staff power was unquestioned in the implementation of the intervention, and there was agreement that there was little impact from the exercise part. While there were unexpected outcomes such as the development of a Wii tournament after a Wii console was acquired for the exercise part of the intervention, and people from other group homes visited the study home, the conclusion was the intervention had a limited impact and may have been more successful if people with learning disabilities were seen as active participants:

> This would stimulate personal responsibility and motivate them to implement their new knowledge in everyday life. Further, it would challenge staff to provide tools that provide independence.
>
> *(Umb Carlsson 2021 p226)*

At this late stage of the book, I hope readers will forgive any eye-rolling seeping through my body to my fingertips and words I am typing. I do not want to single-out individual studies or authors and know my work over the past 15 years does not bear scrutiny. What I want to do though is highlight the limitations in so much work in this area, flawed research designs that lack robustness and the involvement of people with learning disabilities, and the wider lack of thought, knowledge or understanding these studies unintentionally highlight. The introduction of Wii fitness into people's lives seems to be an opportunity to introduce fun, movement and activity that should not need a research project to generate. Indeed, evidence suggests use of the Wii drops off when it is used as part of a physiotherapy programme (Chung et al 2016).

In a co-produced study about eating and living well, Doherty et al (2020) found participants were frustrated by the lack of accessible information around healthy eating, unmet training needs of support staff and family carers and a lack of money. They also found inequities in access to weight management services which can be added to the other support services people with learning disabilities are excluded from, discussed in previous chapters. The authors conclude better collaborative working is needed between people, support staff, general practitioners and service commissioners.

Mothers have described the delicate balance of trying to ensure their adult daughter or son eats well in group homes without annoying support staff. This includes making the food for their relative or using humour to try to point out that the diet being offered is limited (Adolfsson et al 2024). In Sweden, Registered Dieticians are supposed to work with people with learning disabilities to help with nutritional issues; however, it has been found these professionals do not have much knowledge of people with learning disabilities living in group homes, and tensions around choice and autonomy can remain (Adolfsson et al. 2019, Adolfsson et al 2024).

In Australia, another formalised intervention, the Food and Lifestyle Information Programme (FLIP) was designed with people with learning disabilities and is currently being evaluated (Asher et al 2024). Interestingly, there were some contradictions between the views of support workers and people with learning disabilities. For example, support workers thought it was easier for everyone to cook the same dish rather than different dishes to share while participants with learning disabilities preferred the opportunity to cook different dishes, bringing into consideration the shared and social aspect of the activity, agency and creativity.

An intervention developed in the United States demonstrated the potential to improve nutrition by focusing on improving available food (Humphries et al 2009). Preliminary work before the intervention was designed showed staff training was not an option due to low staff retention and the weight of existing training requirements. There are clear implications here for the efficacy of an evidence base for which staff training is the go-to recommendation. Indeed, Sirotkin (2024 p140) found support staff who perceived training to be pointless and irrelevant to practice would do the minimum to comply with formal training requirements and it became a tick box exercise. One participant, for example, described how "... it's in one ear and out the other. Or I can trot it out but I can't do it".

Attitudes, facilitating health diets, cooking skills and dietary knowledge should be taken into consideration when planning dietary interventions (Røstad-Tollefsen et al 2021). Staff should be supported to be positive and motivated in their work, people will need support in planning healthy meals and learning practical cooking skills. A small cluster randomised control trial involved monthly dietary lessons for people with learning disabilities and support staff, and nudges which included posters of fruit and small gifts. The intervention group reduced their waist circumference and improved their blood parameters and healthy eating habits (Røstad-Tollefsen et al 2023). This is promising, the authors conclude, although a larger trial is needed to further test the findings.

A more organic attempt to introduce these pleasures into people's lives was a small pilot study in New Jersey, the United States, which introduced vegetable gardens and cooking classes into group homes to see if these encouraged people with learning disabilities to eat more healthily (LoBuono et al 2024). The cooking classes were well received though the gardens did not get used. Cross-disciplinary students were involved in delivering the lessons and this provided them with a useful, immersive experience. Finally, an evaluation of an assistive technology device 'Bestic' in Sweden found that the novelty of the robot wore off quite quickly and participants preferred to be supported to eat (Dag et al 2017). This was in part because of the time it took to use the device which meant the food got cold.

This brief overview of some of what we know about food and eating in relation to people with learning disabilities has proved to be instructive in terms of highlighting and developing some key issues which I return to in the final section. It has also generated evidence that adding further training to a precarious workforce already burdened by training requirements is problematic. Before we head to the final section, I want to take a detour to discuss a key finding of the *Flourishing Lives* project. This may help to gently disentangle us from the pervasive noise, nonsense and sometimes absurdity that shrouds this area.

10 Minutes of Britney

Medical students have been encouraged to "make strange" and critically question and challenge systemic issues and power relationships in their work (Kumagai and Wear 2014). We saw, in Chapter 2, how DasGuptas (2008) calls for narrative humility which involves a determined consideration of and listening to others. People are, however, comprehensively made strange across their lives from when they first receive the label of learning disabilities. Deliberately and reflectively 'making strange' cannot work in this context, instead, we need to 'unstrange' people and remove the phobic conditions that cause people without learning disabilities to feel fear and/or revulsion.

Our *Flourishing Lives* project unexpectedly provided one mechanism to do this. After fieldwork which involved interviews and focus groups with 50 people with learning disabilities and 28 family carers (Ryan and O'Brien 2024), we held an online learning community of people with learning disabilities, support workers, family carers and academics. The six two-hour online sessions, each held three times to enable participation, covered key findings from the fieldwork; the importance of confidence, belonging and thinking ahead. The aim of the learning community was to think about how to operationalise the importance of having opportunities to do things we value. In the fifth session, we introduced Sen's Capability Approach (2009) which underpinned the project. The technical terms Sen uses, not least the name of the approach, generated a challenge in trying to make his ideas digestible. We finally decided on using an illustration of a woman, Carla, with three thought bubbles above her head. These had images of drinking tea, walking the dog and cooking and represented the things Carla valued. To her side was her weekly planner which showed bowling, the cinema, McDonalds and cleaning. Using this image, we were able to demonstrate that while Carla had a full week in terms of activities, she was not doing anything she valued. This image generated lightbulb moments among participants. In particular, Cassandra, a support worker, talked about how important listening to Britney Spears is to her:

> I just find if I'm having a particularly stressful day [...] or I've got a lot to think about, I put the music on and after about 3 or 4 minutes find myself humming

> and singing along to it. So it must take my mind off it subconsciously, I always feel a bit better I suppose. [unpublished data extract]

She then made the link between her enjoyment of Britney and the importance of someone she supported to have the wind on his face.

> there's a gentleman who likes to sit outside with the wind. So how do I capture that and make sure that's built in, given the importance and praise that it's worth. 10 minutes out there is worth just as much as going to see Britney Spears to me. So it's how that is highlighted and the importance [...] and it's how we show and demonstrate those little importances to us all. [unpublished data extract]

Cassandra's final point about how we note the small importances that matter to all of us was a breakthrough in the project as it seemed to clear away debris and detritus and allow us to clearly see how connected we all are. '10 Minutes of Britney' was used to share the project findings with a range of audiences, including NHS England, the CQC, Bradford City Council and an NHS Trust in the north of England in a tour of one-hour sessions led by self-advocates Beth Richards and Rebecca Spalding and family carers, Angeli Vaid and Alan Spalding. We collected examples of '10 Minutes of Britney' from attendees and found they were largely all free and easy to organise. For example, having a cup of tea in a favourite mug in the morning, walking the dog, sitting in the garden, singing in the kitchen, cooking, spending time with family, binge-watching a box set, and running.

What was unexpected was how '10 Minutes of Britney' impacted team members. It created space for us all to think about the small things we take for granted and yet give us so much contentment. It was only when we imagined our '10 minutes' being denied that the importance of these moments became clear. We concluded, methodological innovation is needed to understand what people value and what it might take to achieve this (Ryan and O'Brien 2024).

Person-centred planning, a stalwart of social care in the UK, possibly had a similar original foundation and yet has been bureaucratised and transformed into tickbox exercises. It has been argued person-centred planning can reproduce and reinforce the dehumanisation of people with learning disabilities as it falls to individual staff members who may lack the capacity to prioritise people's preferences to operationalise it (Sirotkin 2024). It is also aimed at people with learning disabilities thereby delineating people as a specific group which is inherently problematic. No 'intervention' will work while the supporting mechanisms simply reinforce differences between 'us' and 'them'. We need to remove these distinctions. Thinking about cooking as '10 minutes of Britney' rather than an intervention seems so much simpler and possible. Being supported to cook good food and sharing that food with people you know should not be something extraordinary.

Postscript: closing thoughts

In April 2024, in the Jermyn Street Theatre, just off Piccadilly Circus in central London, *Laughing Boy*, an adaptation of my book (Ryan 2017) opened to a full house. Steve Unwin, director and writer, created an extraordinary and literally breathtaking 90 minutes of laughter, tears, pin drop moments of quiet, parody and overwhelming emotion. The cast of seven actors and creative team exemplified narrative humility in listening to our family during the development of the production and rehearsals, and trying to understand our lives with Connor. Steve's son, Joey, who is just a bit younger than Connor has learning disabilities and epilepsy, and another cast member has a sister with learning disabilities. They all came to the production with open hearts, curiosity and a determination to do Connor and our family, justice.

One of the most compelling parts of the play was the projection of a photo montage onto the back of the stage. It included photos of people with learning disabilities who died preventable deaths since Connor's death in 2013. Seeing these beautiful, interesting, quirky faces was shocking and the audience reactions were so visible and audible they were often noted in the daily show reports. The play-run over six weeks generated a rare moment in which audience members enjoyed getting to know Connor and his fascination with London buses and social justice, laughed with him, and felt shock and outrage at what happened to him, and so many other people labelled with learning disabilities. I offer this brief interlude to show how different we can, as a society, act and be. The loose collective I refer to across this book is in reality a small and shifting number of people who wield considerable and rarely challenged power. I suspect many people who know little about the lives of people with learning disabilities would be genuinely horrified to find out how people are treated and the consequence of this treatment. *Laughing Boy* demonstrated this with compelling heart and emotion.

Moving on to think about endings. … We have across this journey explored landscapes of healthcare, love and intimacy, pregnancy and childbirth, housing, employment, food and eating which have generated discrete and overlapping challenges and issues. There is little space, will or interest in supporting people with learning disabilities to lead growing and flourishing lives, and often little or no consideration of people as human. At the same time, people with learning disabilities can deny, deflect and subvert what is thrown at them, repeatedly, from different directions, and remain resourceful, resilient and sometimes ebullient.

So where have we got to?

People with learning disabilities love and are loved, care and contribute in ways that are often not recognised or noticed. People may not be listened to in whatever form or shape the telling may take, and there is a gap in collective resources to be able to articulate or understand what it is like to live in the world as a person labelled with learning disabilities. People experience micro-aggressions and acts of violence across their often-shortened lifetimes which can take the form of disrespect, cruelty, the destruction of dignity making, inclusion phobia, a lack of access to appropriate, timely and effective health and social care, and disproportionate levels of surveillance, scrutiny and limitations on what is possible. The impact of these repeated and myriad injustices on the health and well-being of people is substantial and can contribute to premature death. I argue this constitutes social murder as the conditions for these deaths are repeatedly documented and overwhelmingly ignored.

People are forced into material conditions in which they cannot continue to live and yet, as we have seen across this book, these conditions continue untroubled, often without recognition or meaningful acknowledgement. Grover (2019), in his analysis of 'austerity' social security policy, follows Engels' (1993 [1845] interpretation that social murder is an act of omission rather than commission, while not excusing the avoidable consequences of this policy. I struggle to think how it is possible to consider omission in relation to the deaths of people with learning disabilities given the weight of evidence laid out on these pages.

Norrie (2018), discussing the devastating Grenfell Tower fire in London in 2017, highlights the challenges in naming certain acts as criminal because they can be carried out by those at the centre of the community. I am reminded of Mohamed (2024 p4) describing her incredulity and distress as a doctoral student at having to produce a catalogue of colonial-based violences experienced by Black South Africans to disrupt "overbearing epistemologies of ignorance". She constantly questioned 'surely they know?' The fingerprints of the judicial system are on the death certificates of those who died as an outcome of the closure of the Life Esidemeni institution, alongside the Gauteng health officials (Ferlito and Dhai 2018 p156). Evidence of social murder is not hidden and numerous fingerprints are on countless death certificates. As I outlined in Chapter 1, evidence is recorded in public inquiries, reports, research publications, coroners' reports, court judgements and captured, sometimes implicitly, within published research.

Raphael et al (2022 p142), thinking about persistent health inequalities in Canada, ask if anger and polemic is an effective strategy to enable us to move beyond the lack of effective action as "the ultimate goal is addressing the living and working conditions that first sicken and then kill". I do not know the answer to this, although I have been mindful of not leaning towards polemic in writing this book (anger and outrage is a given). The focus on the lives of people with learning disabilities appears to involve a more pedestrian discounting embedded in assumptions, and the associated epistemic and moral failings in simply not knowing enough or caring enough to pay attention. This can be seen by the enduring and typically unquestioned use of offensive language such as 'idiot' and 'moron' while historic terms used in relation to other marginalised groups are seen as taboo (Rix 2023).

People with learning disabilities consistently experience and endure poor practice, absurdities and deceit which breach human rights and professional practice. A loose and shifting collective of social actors, including politicians, social care, health and other professionals, providers, support workers and sometimes family carers, actively sustain this through wilful or unintentional ignorance. Whether deliberate or underpinned by well-meaning intentions is not relevant; neither is acceptable and, given the positions held by many in this collective, unjust. Goodey (2017) would possibly describe this collective as phobic. To paraphrase Don Quixote (Cervantes 2016), there is considerable jousting at windmills here in search of imaginary monsters, alongside self-interest and the cementing of careers. We could imagine health and social care professionals form part of Goffman's 'wise', and indeed some do. However, the strength of embedded prejudices, deceit and associated ignorance among those who should know better remains a serious issue.

The nimbleness and labour around the operation of this deceit is substantial. We have seen how sterilisation is proposed for people who are deemed to lack capacity, are not able to consent to intimate relations or are unable to raise a child. People are prescribed medication without a formal diagnosis of mental ill-health and may not receive an annual health check and medication review because they are not flagged on the GP register. I described in Chapter 2 how this involves incompetence or wilful participation in a selective and spurious use of 'medical expertise' on the part of health professionals. These actions are apparent across health and social care, regulatory and legal practices. There is an absence of challenge in relation to clear human rights breaches, and the countless moral bystanders are arguably as culpable as those who are directly implicated.

We saw in Chapter 3 the description of the soft power of the disability service where the rules are simply made up (Feely 2016). This can be illustrated by shifting landscapes of surveillance practices; switched on full in relation to sex and intimacy and quietly flipped off in death (unless there is an event of social murder on an unprecedented level such as the Esidemeni scandal (Capri et al 2018)). Mandatory and supposedly robust processes and procedures to protect people, such as the legal system, regulatory processes and safeguarding procedures remain silent. Indeed, safeguarding, alongside other eugenic practices, can be used to prevent people from having opportunities most people take for granted. On the rare occasion action is taken, for example, after the publication of the Mazar's review discussed in Chapter 2, the subsequent learning, in this instance around preventable deaths, is used to improve the lives of the mainstream population, leaving the lives of people with learning disabilities untouched. There is an unflinching, unapologetic and unacknowledged taking from enduring pain and devastation.

We saw in Chapter 3 how family court systems in Iceland and Canada contain documented falsehoods and embellishment in relation to parents with learning disabilities (Pacheco et al 2024, Rice and Sigurjónsdóttir 2018). For Rice and Sigurjónsdóttir (2018), this involves IQ overshadowing, practices that are no doubt replicated across various settings and jurisdictions. I am beginning to question the use of the term diagnostic overshadowing. Mohamed (2024) highlights how academics can turn the cruelty inflicted on people into meaningless abstraction and diagnostic overshadowing is arguably used to account for or excuse violences that should generate action and redress. Instead, the violence is folded into the fabric of oppression and smoothed away.

Support workers can play a crucial role in the happiness and wellbeing of people with learning disabilities and yet support work is an undervalued and poorly supported job. Support staff may be expected to undertake numerous training courses while the core strand of the role – understanding what people value, their '10 Minutes of Britney' and recognising the people with learning disabilities are human – is overlooked. Spending time getting to know people and what is important to them is undervalued and deprioritised in favour of what are seen as functional tasks like feeding (Sirotkin 2024). This absence of acknowledged personhood generates a swathe of restrictions, human rights abuses and subsequently impoverished lives. There is a discernable poignancy around reported interactions between people and their support staff apparent in the earlier discussion around food and eating. It is a dehumanising act to deliberately watch someone eat and then eat separately. The discomfort for some staff is clear alongside staff who intentionally refuse to eat with or even use the same utensils as the people they support. Given the risible social networks people with learning disabilities can have, the distance between staff and the people they support generated by incomprehensible rules and processes is cruel. It should not be difficult to recruit staff with similar interests as the person being supported to enable shared enjoyment of activities. As we found in *Flourishing Lives*, it is not a costly exercise to widen our lives.

We largely know what we know about the lives of people with learning disabilities through personal experiences or research findings. People with learning disabilities are excluded from other areas of life such as being part of, or even seen in, their local community and are rarely represented in literature, film, television or social media other than in simplistic and stereotypical ways. A rare counter example is, of course, the *Laughing Boy* production mentioned above. The role of researchers is therefore crucial and yet not fully recognised or discussed (although the work of, for example, Thomas 2024 and Mohamed 2024, and others are redressing this). Researchers can uncritically use oppressive language while failing to understand people's lives through not working with them. Not seeing people with learning disabilities as human inevitably leads to distorted scholarship and the generation of 'dodgy data' which loop back to underpin and seemingly substantiate the assumptions upon which the research is based.

Research practice should involve upholding human rights, critically examining and calling out injustices. In areas of hermeneutical and testimonial injustices, research practice is a form of witnessing. I have demonstrated across this book examples of human rights breaches written into research without reflection or comment. We saw in Chapter 2 how research practice excluded people with learning disabilities from thousands of government funded projects in England. We also saw with considerable clarity in Chapter 1 how disability studies, critical or otherwise, is complicit in this oppression. It is saddening to see the ease with which marginalised groups can, in turn, enact violences on other marginalised groups. The awkward shunning of people labelled with learning disabilities, the lack of consideration or solidarity among disability study scholars again reveals so much that is ignored.

Research practice can also illuminate and nudge, for example, support staff or health and social care professionals to think more generatively as we saw in Chapter 3 when support staff expressed surprise during research interviews at recognising the lack of consideration about aspects of people's lives such as love and intimate relationships. Research can be a form of activism in ways that demands more attention. At the same time, we need more academic courage and clarity to call out poor practice, to challenge dodgy scholarship, to enable and support researchers to fully involve people in research and to stop being part of the problem.

We need to work together, to carefully listen to people with learning disabilities, in the various ways described across this book and draw on strong allies, the own and the wise, who can help support people's imaginaries and freedoms. The self-advocacy movement while fragmented and under-resourced provides evidence of clear thinking and strong activism, and it is a salutary reminder that the work of these groups can involve advocating for the lives of others. My Life My Choice, discussed in Chapter 2, for example, donates money to other charitable causes (see https://mylifemychoice.org.uk/). In turn, those who are part of the collective, who are jousting at windmills, need to think about what it is they really fear and the sometimes death making consequences (Wolfensberger 1987) of their actions. A strength of the own and the wise is the inherently open and welcoming groupings; as evidenced by the pockets of brilliance recalled by family members sometimes years later (Ryan 2018).

Concluding thoughts

The process of writing this book has generated many emotions, largely dominated by sadness, and countless moments of incredulity. I cannot imagine or even begin to articulate the (un-grievable) pain, glimpses into the lives and experiences of people presented across these pages touch upon. Alongside this 'formal' record are emails and messages I receive from family members documenting devastating accounts of social murder. Actual stories about real people. Much loved family members tossed into Kanner's human waste bin eighty or so years on. While finishing this chapter, I received an email from a mother about a young man who died after repeatedly banging his head while held in a short-term unit for 10 days. She said:

> People who are this sensitive are actually really beautiful in their own way, need our support but they do not get it.

This book is dominated by the voices and words of non-disabled people, with my own as a foghorn. We scatter pellets of so-called knowledge without fully understanding or listening to people with learning disabilities. Testimonial injustice is deeply felt as not only are people ignored and unheard, their experiences, feelings, perceptions and knowledge are brutally discounted. In Chapter 1, I discussed how the continuing existence of people with learning disabilities has been described as astounding (Goodley 2023) and the threat of being cast as human waste, of being disposable, continues to loom large. Recognising and acknowledging this optimistic and complicating resilience (Goodley 2005) is important, as people continue to live, love and labour.

I have presented a harrowing account of the absurd and contrary ways people are treated and forced to lead their lives. Empty promises of supporting autonomy and choice, a polished ignoring of human rights abuses despite a comprehensive historic evidence base of abuse, trauma and brutality. The concept of epistemic injustice, while offering important insights and considerations, does not fully reach the spot here. The careful plotting of inclusion phobia leaves unanswered questions over 'and?' Other theoretical accounts such as Altermark's (2017) meticulous biopolitical analysis offer ways of thinking about, understanding and interpreting while remaining abstracted from the everyday lives of people in the here and now. We have witnessed the brutality and torture of people labelled with learning disabilities for too long now. We can no longer offer our often-problematic research findings, our overly optimistic and repetitive research recommendations and wander off to the next research project.

I have strongly argued that the premature and preventable deaths of people with learning disabilities constitute social murder. We are, as Kittay (2001) argued nearly 25 years ago, shirking our collective responsibility to take care of each other. Collaboration is key in terms of supporting people and positive freedoms, of paying attention to the space around us all. In relation to this, I end by acknowledging the courage and commitment to change demonstrated by the own and the wise; people with learning disabilities, family members, support workers and many other allies. To the shagging in the sensory room and being more than 'just a disability person'.

REFERENCES

Abbas, A. 2010. Incorporating the victim. In *Liberalism and human suffering: Materialist reflections on politics, ethics, and aesthetics*, edited by A. Abbas (pp. 19–43). New York: Palgrave Macmillan US.

Abbott, D. 2015. Love in a cold climate: Changes in the fortunes of LGBT men and women with learning disabilities? *British Journal of Learning Disabilities*, *43*(2), pp.100–105.

Adolfsson, P., Ek, P. and Umb Carlsson, Õ. 2019. Dietitians' challenges when consulting to adults with intellectual disabilities. *Tizard Learning Disability Review*, *24*, pp.153–162.

Adolfsson, P., Mattsson Sydner, Y. and Fjellström, C. 2010. Social aspects of eating events among people with intellectual disability in community living. *Journal of Intellectual and Developmental Disability, 35*(4), pp.259–267.

Adolfsson, P., Umb Carlsson, Õ. and Ek, P. 2024. Significant others' perspectives on experiences of meal-oriented support and diet counselling for adults with intellectual disabilities who live in supported housing. *International Journal of Developmental Disabilities, 70*(3), pp.435–443.

Alcoff, L. 2007. Epistemologies of ignorance. Three types. In *Race and epistemologies of ignorance*, edited by S. Sullivan and N. Tuana (pp.39–57). Albany: State University of New York Press.

Alexandra, P., Angela, H. and Ali, A. 2018. Loneliness in people with intellectual and developmental disorders across the lifespan: A systematic review of prevalence and interventions. *Journal of Applied Research in Intellectual Disabilities, 31*(5), pp.643–658.

Ali, A., Scior, K., Ratti, V., Strydom, A., King, M. and Hassiotis, A. 2013. Discrimination and other barriers to accessing health care: perspectives of patients with mild and moderate intellectual disability and their carers. *PloS One, 8*(8), p.e70855.

Almalky, H.A., 2020. Employment outcomes for individuals with intellectual and developmental disabilities: A literature review. *Children and Youth Services Review*, *109*, p.104656.

Allen, H. and Fuller, E. 2016. Beyond the feeble mind: Foregrounding the personhood of inmates with significant intellectual disabilities in the era of institutionalization. *Disability Studies Quarterly, 36*(2), n.p.

Altermark, N. 2017. *Citizenship inclusion and intellectual disability: Biopolitics post-institutionalisation*. London: Routledge.

AM, S. 2022. Notions of sexuality: An analysis of the interplays of gender and care among adults with intellectual disabilities in Kerala. *Journal of Gender Studies, 31*(7), pp.863–873.

Amelink, Q., Roozen, S., Leistikow, I. and Weenink, J.W. 2021. Sexual abuse of people with intellectual disabilities in residential settings: A 3-year analysis of incidents reported to the Dutch Health and Youth Care Inspectorate. *BMJ Open, 11*(12), p.e053317.

Amy, J.J. and Rowlands, S. 2018. Legalised non-consensual sterilisation–eugenics put into practice before 1945, and the aftermath. Part 1: USA, Japan, Canada and Mexico. *The European Journal of Contraception & Reproductive Health Care, 23*(2), pp.121–129.

Anders, P.L. and Davis, E.L. 2010. Oral health of patients with intellectual disabilities: A systematic review. *Special Care in Dentistry, 30*(3), pp.110–117.

Anderson, E. 2012. Epistemic justice as a virtue of social institutions. *Social Epistemology, 26*(2), pp.163–173.

Anderson, S. and Bigby, C., 2017. Self-advocacy as a means to positive identities for people with intellectual disability:'We just help them, be them really'. *Journal of Applied Research in Intellectual Disabilities*, 30(1), pp.109-120.

Anderson, L.L., Humphries, K., McDermott, S., Marks, B., Sisirak, J. and Larson, S. 2013. The state of the science of health and wellness for adults with intellectual and developmental disabilities. *Intellectual and Developmental Disabilities, 51*(5), pp.385–398.

Anderson, R.J., Keagan-Bull, R., Giles, J. and Tuffrey-Wijne, I. 2023. "My name on the door by the Professor's name": The process of recruiting a researcher with a learning disability at a UK university. *British Journal of Learning Disabilities, 51*(3), pp.460–468.

Annison, J.E. 2000. Towards a clearer understanding of the meaning of "home". *Journal of Intellectual and Developmental Disability, 25*(4), pp.251–262.

Appelgren, M., Bahtsevani, C., Persson, K. and Borglin, G. 2018. Nurses' experiences of caring for patients with intellectual developmental disorders: A systematic review using a meta-ethnographic approach. *BMC Nursing, 17*, pp.1–19.

Appolloni, L. and D'Alessandro, D. 2021. Housing spaces in nine European countries: A comparison of dimensional requirements. *International Journal of Environmental Research and Public Health, 18*, 4278.

Ash, A. 2016. *Whistleblowing and ethics in health and social care*. London: Jessica Kingsley Publishers.

Asher, R.C., Shrewsbury, V.A., Innes, B., Fitzpatrick, A., Simmonds, S. and Collins, C.E. 2024. Designing the Food and Lifestyle Information Program (FLIP) culinary nutrition intervention for adults with mild-to-moderate intellectual disability. *Journal of Human Nutrition and Dietetics, 37*(4), pp.1109–1122.

Atuahene, B. 2016. Dignity takings and dignity restoration: Creating a new theoretical framework for understanding involuntary property loss and the remedies required. *Law and Society Inq, 41*(4), pp.796–823.

Aull Davies, C.A. 2007. Food and the social identities of people with learning disabilities. *Disability Studies Quarterly, 27*(3), n.p.

Badcock, E. and Sakellariou, D. 2022. "Treating him … like a piece of meat": Poor communication as a barrier to care for people with learning disabilities. *Disability Studies Quarterly*, *42*(1), n.p.

Bahner, J. 2020. Sexual citizenship, disability policy and facilitated sex in Sweden 1. In *The Routledge handbook of disability and sexuality*, edited by R. Shuttleworth and L.R. Mona (pp. 171–184). Oxon: Routledge.

Bahner, J., Gäddman Johansson, R. and Svanelöv, E. 2024. Who counts as a sexual subject? The impact of ableist rhetoric for people with intellectual disability in Sweden. *Sexuality Research and Social Policy, 21*(1), pp.161–176.

Bahner, J., Kulick, D. and Fernández, A.G.S. 2023. The devil is in the details. *Archives of Sexual Behavior, 52*(8), pp.3259–3261.

Bakker-van Gijssel, E.J., Olde Hartman, T.C., Lucassen, P.L., van den Driessen, M.F., Dees, M.K., Assendelft, W.J., et al. 2017. GPs' opinions of health assessment instruments for people with intellectual disabilities: A qualitative study. *British Journal of General Practice, 67*(654), pp.e41–ee8.

Baksh, R.A., Pape, S.E., Smith, J. and Strydom, A. 2021. Understanding inequalities in COVID-19 outcomes following hospital admission for people with intellectual disability compared to the general population: A matched cohort study in the UK. *BMJ Open, 11*(10), p.e052482.

Ball, S.L., Panter, S.G., Redley, M., Proctor, C.A., Byrne, K., Clare, I.C.H. and Holland, A.J. 2012. The extent and nature of need for mealtime support among adults with intellectual disabilities. *Journal of Intellectual Disability Research, 56*(4), pp.382–401.

Bambra, C., Gibson, M., Sowden, A., Wright, K., Whitehead, M. and Petticrew, M. 2010. Tackling the wider social determinants of health and health inequalities: Evidence from systematic reviews. *Journal of Epidemiology & Community Health, 64*(4), pp.284–291.

Barger, E., Wacker, J., Macy, R., Parish, S. 2009. Sexual assault prevention for women with intellectual disabilities: A critical review of the evidence. *Intellectual and Developmental Disabilities, 47*, pp.249–262.

Bates, C., Terry, L. and Popple, K. 2017. The importance of romantic love to people with learning disabilities. *British Journal of Learning Disabilities, 45*(1), pp.64–72.

Berger, J. 2019. Rethink: Agency, theory and politics in disability studies. In *Manifestos for the future of critical disability studies* (Vol. 1), edited by K. Ellis, R. Garland-Thomson, M. Kent and R. Robertson (pp. 209–216). Oxon: Routledge.

Bigby, C. and Fyffe, C. 2009. Achieving their own lives: The implementation of individualised funding for people with intellectual disability. *Proceedings of the third annual roundtable on intellectual disability policy. Melbourne: La Trobe University.*

Bindmans. 2025. www.bindmans.com/news-insights/news/justice-for-ap-oxford-health-nhs-foundation-trust-pays-damages-following-detention-and-seclusion-of-man-with-learning-disabilities-and-autism-for-340-days/. Retrieved 16 February 2025.

Blood, L., Ribenfors, F., Hatton, C. and Marriott, A. 2024. Moving house: How much choice do people with learning disabilities have about where they live?. *British Journal of Learning Disabilities*, *52*(1), pp.140–149.

Bloom, O. and Morison, T. 2024. Supporting intellectually disabled women's sexual and reproductive health and rights: A qualitative study with support workers in Aotearoa New Zealand. *Women's Reproductive Health, 11*(2), pp.396–416.

Borras, A.M. and Mohamed, F.A. 2020. Health inequities and the shifting paradigms of food security, food insecurity, and food sovereignty. *International Journal of Health Services, 50*(3), pp.299–313.

Bould, E., Bigby, C., Bennett, P.C. and Howell, T.J. 2018. "More people talk to you when you have a dog" – Dogs as catalysts for social inclusion of people with intellectual disabilities. *Journal of Intellectual Disability Research*, *62*(10), pp.833–841.

Bouzas, S., Martínez-Lemos, R.I. and Ayan, C. 2019. Effects of exercise on the physical fitness level of adults with intellectual disability: A systematic review. *Disability and Rehabilitation, 41*(26), pp.3118–3140.

Bowey, L. and McGlaughlin, A. 2007. Older carers of adults with a learning disability confront the future: Issues and preferences in planning. *British Journal of Social Work, 37*(1), pp.39–54.

Bradbury-Jones, C., Rattray, J., Jones, M. and MacGillivray, S. 2013. Promoting the health, safety and welfare of adults with learning disabilities in acute care settings: A structured literature review. *Journal of Clinical Nursing, 22*(11-12), pp.1497–1509.

Braidotti, R. 2012. "Becoming-world". In *After cosmopolitanism*, edited by R. Braidotti, P. Hanafin and B. Blaagaard (pp. 8–27). Routledge.

Brison, S.J. 2021. Valuing the lives of people with profound intellectual disabilities. *Philosophical Topics, 49*(1), pp.99–122.

Brookes, N., Palmer, S., Collins, G. and Callaghan, L. 2024. Supporting people to live well: A multimethod study of Shared Lives (adult placement). *British Journal of Learning Disabilities*, *52*(1), pp.131–139.

Brown, M., Harry, M. and Mahoney, K. 2018a. "It's like two roles we're playing": Parent perspectives on navigating self-directed service programs with adult children with intellectual and/or developmental disabilities. *Journal of Policy and Practice in Intellectual Disabilities*, *15*(4), pp.350–358.

Brown, M. and McCann, E. 2018. Sexuality issues and the voices of adults with intellectual disabilities: A systematic review of the literature. *Research in Developmental Disabilities, 74*, pp. 124–138.

Burgard, S.A., Seefeldt, K.S. and Zelner, S. 2012. Housing instability and health: Findings from the Michigan Recession and Recovery Study. *Social Science & Medicine, 75*(12), pp.2215–2224.

Butler, I. and Drakeford, M. 2005. *Scandal, social policy and social welfare.* Bristol University Press.

Byrne, G. 2018. Prevalence and psychological sequelae of sexual abuse among individuals with an intellectual disability: A review of the recent literature. *Journal of Intellectual Disabilities*, *22*(3), pp.294–310.

Callaghan, L., Brookes, N. and Palmer, S. 2017. Older people receiving family-based support in the community: A survey of quality of life among users of 'Shared Lives' in England. *Health & Social Care in the Community, 25*(5), pp.1655–1666.

Callow, E., Tahir, M. and Feldman, M. 2017. Judicial reliance on parental IQ in appellate-level child welfare cases involving parents with intellectual and developmental disabilities. *Journal of Applied Research in Intellectual Disabilities, 30*(3), pp.553–562.

Caltabiano, P., Bailie, J., Laycock, A., Shea, B., Dykgraaf, S.H., Lennox, N., Ekanayake, K. and Bailie, R. 2024. Identifying barriers and facilitators to primary care practitioners implementing health assessments for people with intellectual disability: A Theoretical Domains Framework-informed scoping review. *Implementation Science Communication, 5*(1), p. 39.

Campbell, M. 2017. Disabilities and sexual expression: A review of the literature. *Sociology Compass, 11*(9), pp.1–19.

Capasso, L. and D'Alessandro, D. 2021. Housing and health: Here we go again. *International Journal of Environmental Research and Public Health*, *18*(22), p.12060.

Capri, C., Watermeyer, B., Mckenzie, J. and Coetzee, O. 2018. Intellectual disability in the Esidimeni tragedy: Silent deaths. *SAMJ: South African Medical Journal, 108*(3), pp.153–154.

Carel, H. and Kidd, I.J. 2021. Institutional opacity, epistemic vulnerability, and institutional testimonial justice. *International Journal of Philosophical Studies, 29*(4) pp.473–496.

Carey, A. 2009. *On the margins of citizenship: Intellectual disability and civil rights in twentieth-century America.* Temple University Press.

Carey, I.M., Hosking, F.J., Harris, T., De Wilde, S., Beighton, C. and Cook, D.G. 2017. An evaluation of the effectiveness of annual health checks and quality of health care for adults with intellectual disability: An observational study using a primary care database. *Health Services and Delivery Research, 5*(25), pp.1–170.

Carlson, L. 2010. *The faces of intellectual disability: Philosophical reflections.* Bloomington: Indiana UP.

Carter, A., Strnadová, I., Watfern, C., Pebdani, R., Bateson, D., Loblinzk, J., Guy, R., Newman, C. 2021.The sexual and reproductive health and rights of young people with intellectual disability: A scoping review. *Sexuality Research and Social Policy, 19*, pp.372–390.

Cartwright, L., Reid, M., Hammersley, R., Blackburn, C. and Glover, L. 2015. Food choice by people with intellectual disabilities at day centres: A qualitative study. *Journal of Intellectual Disabilities*, *19*(2), pp.103–115.

Casey, A.F. and Rasmussen, R. 2013. Reduction measures and percentage body fat in individuals with intellectual disabilities: A scoping review. *Disability and Health Journal*, *6*(1), pp.2–7.

Cassidy, G., Martin, D.M., Martin, G.H. and Roy, A. 2002. Health checks for people with learning disabilities: Community learning disability teams working with general practitioners and primary health care teams. *Journal of Learning Disabilities, 6*(2), pp.123–136.

Cavanagh, D.E., Caton, S., Rawles, J., Runswick-Cole, K., Hatton, C., Chauhan, U. and Hutchinson, C. 2024. What do people with intellectual disabilities, their family members and paid carers understand about psychotropic medication? A rapid review. *Journal of Applied Research in Intellectual Disabilities*, *37*(5), p.e13283.

Cervantes, M. 2016. *Don Quixote*. Simon and Schuster.

Chadwick, D.D., Jolliffe, J. and Goldbart, J. 2003. Adherence to eating and drinking guidelines for adults with intellectual disabilities and dysphagia. *American Journal on Mental Retardation*, *108*(3), pp.202–211.

Charitou, M., Quayle, E. and Sutherland, A. 2021. Supporting adults with intellectual disabilities with relationships and sex: A systematic review and thematic synthesis of qualitative research with staff. *Sexuality and Disability*, *39*, pp.113–146.

Chen, B.W., Chou, Y.C. and Chi, H.C. 2022. Unpacking the cultural paradox of attentive care for institutionalized people with intellectual disabilities. *Health & Place*, *78*, p.102821.

Chicoine, C., Hickey, E.E., Kirschner, K.L. and Chicoine, B.A. 2022. Ableism at the bedside: People with intellectual disabilities and COVID-19. *The Journal of the American Board of Family Medicine*, *35*(2), pp.390–393.

Chinn, D., Levitan, T., Power, A., Brickley, K. and Ali, S. 2024. What does "feeling at home" mean for adults with intellectual disabilities living in group homes in England? *Journal of Applied Research in Intellectual Disabilities*, *37*(5), e13274. https://doi.org/10.1111/jar.13274

Chong, K., Cheah, K.J. and Manokara, V. 2024. Our lives, our voices: Impact of self-advocacy program on persons with intellectual developmental disability. *Advances in Neurodevelopmental Disorders*, *8*(1), pp.42–63.

Chou, Y.C., Jane Lu, Z.-Y., Chen, B.-W. and Lin, C.-J. 2020. Awareness of sexual rights and empowerment: Quantitative and qualitative evaluation of a sexual health intervention for adults with intellectual disability. *The Journal of Sex Research*, *57*(9), pp.1202–1216.

Chou, Y.C. and Lu, Z.J. 2011. Deciding about sterilisation: Perspectives from women with an intellectual disability and their families. *Journal of Intellectual Disability Research*, 55, pp.63–74.

Chou, Y.C. and Schalock, R.L. 2007. Trends in residential policies and services for people with intellectual disabilities in Taiwan. *Journal of Intellectual Disability Research, 51*(2), pp.135–141.

Christian, L., Stinson, J. and Dotson, L.A. 2001. Staff values regarding the sexual expression of women with developmental disabilities. *Sexuality and Disability, 19*(4), pp.283–291.

Chung, A.M., Harvey, L.A. and Hassett, L.M. 2016. Do people with intellectual disability use Nintendo Wii when placed in their home as part of a physiotherapy program? An observational study. *Disability and Rehabilitation: Assistive Technology, 11*(4), pp.310–315.

Clawson, R., Patterson, A., Fyson, R. and McCarthy, M. 2020. The demographics of forced marriage of people with learning disabilities: Findings from a national database. *The Journal of Adult Protection, 22*(2), pp.59–74.

Clift, A.K., Coupland, C.A.C., Keogh, R.H., et al. 2021. COVID-19 mortality risk in down syndrome: Results from a cohort study of 8 million adults. *Annals of Internal Medicine,174*, pp572–576.

Cluley, V., Fyson, R. and Pilnick, A. 2020. Theorising disability: A practical and representative ontology of learning disability. *Disability & Society, 35*(2), pp.235–257.

Collings, S., Spencer, M., Dew, A. and Dowse, L. 2018. "She was there if I needed to talk or to try and get my point across": Specialist advocacy for parents with intellectual disability in the Australian child protection system. *Australian Journal of Human Rights, 24*(2), pp.162–181.

Commission on Social Determinants of Health. 2008. *Closing the gap in a generation: Health equity through action on the social determinants of health.* Retrieved from Geneva. http://whqlibdoc.who.int/publications/2008/9789241563703_eng.pdf.

Cooper, S.A., McConnachie, A., Allan, L.M., Melville, C., Smiley, E. and Morrison, J. 2011. Neighbourhood deprivation, health inequalities and service access by adults with intellectual disabilities: A cross-sectional study. *Journal of Intellectual Disability Research, 55*(3), pp. 313–23.

Cooper-Moss, N., Umpleby, K., Roberts, C., Garner, C., Edwards, A.H., Ditzel, N., Butt, J., Clark, S., Hatton, C. and Chauhan, U. 2024. Barriers to healthcare for people with a learning disability from ethnic minorities: Perspectives of self-advocates and carers. *British Journal of Learning Disabilities*. [Early view].

Cuypers, M., Schalk, B.W., Boonman, A.J., Naaldenberg, J. and Leusink, G.L. 2022. Cancer-related mortality among people with intellectual disabilities: A nationwide population-based cohort study. *Cancer, 128*(6), pp.1267–1274.

Ćwirynkało, K. and Parchomiuk, M. 2023. Support as described by fathers with intellectual disabilities. *Journal of Applied Research in Intellectual Disabilities, 36*(2), pp.320–332.

Dag, M., Svanelöv, E. and Gustafsson, C. 2017. Experiences of using Bestic, an eating aid for people with intellectual disabilities. *Journal of Intellectual Disabilities, 21*(1), pp.87–98.

Daly, E. and Smith, O. 2022. The role of space and place in learning disabled people's experiences of disablist violence. In *Landscapes of hate*, edited by E. Hall, J. Clayton and C. Donavan (pp.118–137). Bristol University Press.

DasGupta, S. 2008. Narrative humility. *The Lancet, 371*(9617), pp.980–981.

Davy, L. 2019. Between an ethic of care and an ethic of autonomy: Negotiating relational autonomy, disability, and dependency. *Angelaki, 24*(3), pp.101–114.

Daw Srdonovic, B., Hayden, N., Goodley, D., Lawthom, R. and Runswick-Cole, K. 2024. Failing ethnographies as post-qualitative possibilities: Reflections from critical posthumanities and critical disability studies. *Qualitative Research in Psychology*, pp.1–24.

Dean, S., Marshall, J., Whelan, E., Watson, J., Zorbas, C. and Cameron, A.J. 2021. A systematic review of health promotion programs to improve nutrition for people with intellectual disability. *Current Nutrition Reports*, pp.1–12.

Deffew, A., Coughlan, B., Burke, T. and Rogers, E. 2022. Staff member's views and attitudes to supporting people with an intellectual disability: A multi-method investigation of intimate relationships and sexuality. *Journal of Applied Research in Intellectual Disabilities*, *35*, pp.1049–1058.

de Haas, C. 2020. Singing together. In *Belonging for people with profound intellectual and multiple disabilities: Pushing the boundaries of inclusion,* edited by M. Nind and I. Strnadová. Oxford: Routledge.

de Kuijper, G., Hoekstra, P., Visser, F., Scholte, F. A., Penning, C. and Evenhuis, H. 2010. Use of antipsychotic drugs in individuals with intellectual disability (ID) in The Netherlands: Prevalence and reasons for prescription. *Journal of Intellectual Disability Research*, ***54***, pp.659–667.

Denekens, J.P.M., Nys, H. and Stuer, H. 1999. Sterilisation of incompetent mentally handicapped persons: A model for decision making. *Journal of Medical Ethics, 25*, pp.237–241.

Dhai, A. 2018. The Life Esidimeni tragedy: Moral pathology and an ethical crisis. *SAMJ: South African Medical Journal*, *108*(5), pp.382–385.

Dickinson, H. 2017. Individual funding systems: What works?. *Evidence Base: A Journal of Evidence Reviews in Key Policy Areas*, (3), pp.1–18.

Dijker, A., Van Alphen, L., Bos, A., Van den Borne, B. and Curfs, L. 2011. Social integration of people with intellectual disability: Insights from a social psychological research programme. *Journal of Intellectual Disability Research*, *55*(9), pp.885–894.

Disability Rights Commission. 2006. Equal treatment: Closing the gap a formal investigation into physical health inequalities experienced by people with learning disabilities and/or mental health problems. Available at <http://disability-studies.leeds.ac.uk/wp-content/uploads/sites/40/library/DRC-Health-FI-main.pdf> [Accessed 24 July 2024].

Doherty, A.J., Atherton, H., Boland, P., Hastings, R., Hives, L., Hood, K., James-Jenkinson, L., Leavey, R., Randell, E., Reed, J. and Taggart, L. 2020. Barriers and facilitators to primary health care for people with intellectual disabilities and/or autism: An integrative review. *BJGP Open, 4*(3), n.p.

Doherty, A.J., Jones, S.P., Chauhan, U. and Gibson, J.M.E. 2020b. Eating well, living well and weight management: A co-produced semi-qualitative study of barriers and facilitators experienced by adults with intellectual disabilities. *Journal of Intellectual Disabilities*, *24*(2), pp.158–176.

Dohmen, J. 2016. A little of her language: Epistemic injustice and mental disability. *Research Philosophica*, *93*(4), pp.669–691.

Donohoe, M.T. ed., 2012. *Public Health and Social Justice: A Jossey-Bass Reader*. John Wiley & Sons.

Dotson, K., 2014. Conceptualizing epistemic oppression. *Social Epistemology*, 28(2), pp.115–138.

Douglas, M. 1966. *Purity and danger: An analysis of concepts of taboo and pollution*. London: Routledge & K. Paul.

Doyle, A., O'Sullivan, M., Craig, S. and McConkey, R. 2021. People with intellectual disability in Ireland are still dying young. *Journal of Applied Research in Intellectual Disabilities*, *34*(4), pp.1057–1065.

Drife, J.O., Lewis, G., Neilson, J.P., Knight, M., Cooper, G. and Cantwell, R., 2023. *Why mothers died and how their lives are saved: the story of confidential enquiries into maternal deaths*. Cambridge University Press.

Durbin, A., Isaacs, B., Mauer-Vakil, D. et al. 2018. Intellectual disability and homelessness: A synthesis of the literature and discussion of how supportive housing can support wellness for people with intellectual disability. *Current Developmental Disorders Report, 5*, pp.125–131.

Durkheim, E. 1898/1969. Individualism and the intellectuals (translated by Steven Lukes). *Political Studies, 17*(1), pp.14–30.

Easthope, H. 2004. A place called home. *Housing, Theory and Society*, *21*(3), pp.128–138.

Editorial. 1933. Feeble-minded and the future. *The New England Journal of Medicine, 208*, pp. 852–853.

Editorial. 1934. Sterilization and its possible accomplishments. *The New England Journal of Medicine, 211*, pp.379–380.

Eggleton, I., Robertson, S., Ryan, J. and Kober, R. 1999. The impact of employment on the quality of life of people with an intellectual disability. *Journal of Vocational Rehabilitation*, *13*(2), pp.95–107.

Ellenkamp, J.J., Brouwers, E.P., Embregts, P.J., Joosen, M.C. and van Weeghel, J. 2016. Work environment-related factors in obtaining and maintaining work in a competitive employment setting for employees with intellectual disabilities: A systematic review. *Journal of Occupational Rehabilitation*, *26*, pp.56–69.

Emerson, E. 2004. Cluster housing for adults with intellectual disabilities. *Journal of Intellectual & Developmental Disability*, *29*(3), pp.187–197.

Emerson, E. 2021. Inequalities and inequities in the health of people with intellectual disabilities. *Oxford Research Encyclopedia of Global Public Health.* Retrieved 26 November 2024, from https://oxfordre.com/publichealth/view/10.1093/acrefore/9780190632366.001.0001/acrefore-9780190632366-e-326.

Emerson, E. and Hatton, C. 2014. *Health inequalities and people with intellectual disabilities*. Cambridge University Press.

Engels, F. 1993 [1845]. *The condition of the working class in England.* Oxford: Oxford University Press.

FAO, IFAD, UNICEF, WFP and WHO. 2019. The state of food security and nutrition in the world 2019. Safeguarding against economic slowdowns and downturns. Rome: FAO.

FAO and WHO. 2014. Second international conference on nutrition. Conference outcome document: Rome Declaration on Nutrition, 19-21 November. Rome, Italy: Food and Agriculture Organization & World Health Organization.

Feely, M. 2016. Sexual surveillance and control in a community-based intellectual disability service. *Sexualities*, *19*(5-6), pp.725–750.

Felce, D., Perry, J., Romeo, R., Robertson, J., Meek, A., Emerson, E. and Knapp, M, 2008. Outcomes and costs of community living: semi-independent living and fully staffed group homes. *American Journal on Mental Retardation*, *113*(2), pp.87-101.

Ferlito, B.A. and Dhai, A. 2018. The Life Esidimeni tragedy: The courts are also to blame. *South African Medical Journal*, *108*(3), pp.155–156.

Flannery, K.A. and Wisner-Carlson, R. 2020. Autism and education. Child and Adolescent Psychiatric Clinics, 29(2), pp.319-343.

Flynn, M. and Citarella, V. 2013. Winterbourne View Hospital: A glimpse of the legacy. *The Journal of Adult Protection, 15*(4), pp.173–181.

Flynn, S., Hatton, C. and Coronavirus and People with Learning Disabilities Study Team. 2021. Health and social care access for adults with learning disabilities across the UK during the COVID-19 pandemic in 2020. *Tizard Learning Disability Review, 26*(3), pp.174–179.

Flynn, S., Hatton, C., Hastings, R.P., Hayden, N., Caton, S., Heslop, P., Jahoda, A., Todd, S., Oloidi, E., Beyer, S. and Mulhall, P. 2022. Access to and use of health and social care services for people with learning disabilities during COVID-19: A longitudinal study. *Tizard Learning Disability Review, 27*(1), pp.57–66.

Folch, A., Salvador-Carulla, L., Vicens, P., Cortés, M.J., Irazábal, M., Muñoz, S., Rovira, L., Orejuela, C., González, J.A. and Martínez-Leal, R. 2019. Health indicators in intellectual developmental disorders: The key findings of the POMONA-ESP project. *Journal of Applied Research in Intellectual Disabilities, 32*, pp.23–34.

Fricker, M. 2007. *Epistemic injustice: Power and the ethics of knowing*. New York: Oxford University Press.

Fulford, C. and Cobigo, V. 2018. Friendships and intimate relationships among people with intellectual disabilities: A thematic synthesis. *Journal of Applied Research in Intellectual Disabilities, 31*(1), pp.e18–e35.

Galtung, J. 1973. "The limits to growth" and class politics. *Journal of Peace Research, 10*(1-2), pp.101–114.

García-Largo, L.M., Martí-Agustí, G., Martin-Fumadó, C. and Gómez-Durán, E.L. 2020. Intellectual disability rates among male prison inmates. *International Journal of Law and Psychiatry, 70*, p.101566.

Garland-Thomson, R. 2011. Misfits: A feminist materialist disability concept. *Hypatia, 26*(3), pp.591–609.

Garland-Thomson, R. 2014. The story of my work: How I became disabled. *Disability Studies Quarterly, 34*(2), n.p.

Garland-Thomson, R. 2019. Critical disability studies: A knowledge manifesto. In *Manifestos for the future of critical disability studies*, edited by K. Ellis, R. Garland-Thomson, M. Kent and R. Robertson (pp. 11–19). Routledge.

Garrels, V. and Sigstad, H.M.H. 2021. Employment for persons with intellectual disability in the Nordic countries: A scoping review. *Journal of Applied Research in Intellectual Disabilities, 34*, pp.993–1007.

Gast, D.A., de Wit, G.L., van Hoof, A., de Vries, J.H., van Hemert, B., Didden, R. and Giltay, E.J. 2022. Diet quality among people with intellectual disabilities and borderline intellectual functioning. *Journal of Applied Research in Intellectual Disabilities, 35*(2), pp.488–494.

Gerschick, T.J. and Stevens, J.D. 2016. Invisibility, visibility, vilification, and near silence: The framing of disability in the early years of the American Sociological Society. In *Sociology looking at disability: What did we know and when did we know it*, edited by S.E. Green and S.N. Barnartt (Vol. 9, pp. 1–27). Emerald Group Publishing Limited.

Gilmore, L. and L. Malcolm. 2014. "Best for everyone concerned" or "only as a last resort"? Views of Australian doctors about sterilisation of men and women with intellectual disability. *Journal of Intellectual & Developmental Disability, 39*(2), pp.177–187.

Ginn, H.G. 2022. Securing sexual justice for people with intellectual disability: A systematic review and critical appraisal of research recommendations. *Journal of Applied Research in Intellectual Disabilities, 35*(4), pp.921–934.

Gjertsen, H.G. Hardonk and Ineland J. 2021. Work inclusion for people with intellectual disabilities in three Nordic countries: The current policy and challenges. *Scandinavian Journal of Disability Research, 23*(1), pp.360–370.

Glasby, J., Miller, R., Glasby, A.M., Ince, R. and Konteh, F. 2024. "Why are we stuck in hospital?" Barriers to people with learning disabilities/autistic people leaving "long-stay" hospital: A mixed methods study. *Health and Social Care Delivery Research, 12*(3), pp.1–119.

Glaser, W. and Deane, K. 1999. Normalisation in an abnormal world: A study of prisoners with an intellectual disability. *International Journal of Offender Therapy and Comparative Criminology, 43*(3), pp.338–356.

Glover, G., Williams, R., Branford, D., Avery, R., Chauhan, U., Hoghton, M. and Bernard, S. 2015. *Prescribing of psychotropic drugs to people with learning disabilities and/or autism by general practitioners in England*. Public Health England. PHE standard publication template (uclan.ac.uk).

Goffman, E. 1963. *Stigma: Notes on the management of spoiled identity*. New York: Simon and Schuster.

Goli, S., Noroozi, M. and Salehi, M., 2020. Parental experiences about the sexual and reproductive health of adolescent girls with intellectual disability: A qualitative study. *Iranian Journal of Nursing and Midwifery Research, 25*(3), pp.254–259.

Goodey, C.F. 2017. *Learning disability and inclusion phobia: Past, present, future*. Taylor & Francis.

Goodley, D. 2005. Empowerment, self-advocacy and resilience. *Journal of Intellectual Disabilities, 9*(4), pp.333–343.

Goodley, D. 2023. Being human as praxis: For people with learning disabilities. *Subjectivity, 30*(2), pp.167–184.

Goodley, D. and Rapley, M. 2002. Changing the subject: Postmodernity and people with "learning difficulties". In *Disability/Postmodernity: Embodying Disability Theory*, edited by M. Corker and T. Shakespeare, pp.127–142. Bloomsbury.

Goodwin, D. 2019. NHS inquiries and the problem of culture. *The Political Quarterly, 90*(2), pp.202–209.

Gordon, L.G., Holden, L., Ware, R.S., Taylor, M.T. and Lennox, N. 2012. Comprehensive health assessments for adults with intellectual disability living in the community Weighing up the costs and benefits. *Australian Family Physician, 41*, pp.969–972.

le Goullon, D. 2022. Places to belong, the community experiences of adults with intellectual disabilities. MPhil Thesis, School of Education, The University of Queensland.

Gov.IE. 2023. https://www.gov.ie/en/department-of-housing-local-government-and-heritage/press-releases/implementation-plan-to-deliver-improved-housing-for-disabled-people-is-launched/. Accessed on 17 May 2024.

Gov UK. 2023. www.gov.uk/government/publications/independent-care-education-and-treatment-reviews-government-response-2023/annex-a-dhsc-response-to-individual-recommendations. Accessed on 17 May 2024.

Gréaux, M., Moro, M.F., Kamenov, K., Russell, A.M., Barrett, D. and Cieza, A. 2023. Health equity for persons with disabilities: A global scoping review on barriers and interventions in healthcare services. *International Journal for Equity in Health, 22*(1), pp.236.

Green, S.E., Gerschick, T.J. and Vitullo, M.W. 2017. *American Sociological Association Status Committee on Persons with Disabilities in Sociology Five Year Report to Council*. www.asanet.org/wp-content/uploads/asa_2017_council_report_status_committee_disabilities_final_w_appendices.pdf.

Gregson, N., Randle-Phillips, C. and Hillman, S. 2022. People with intellectual disabilities' experiences of primary care health checks, screenings and GP consultations: A systematic review and meta-ethnography. *International Journal of Developmental Disabilities, 70*(2), pp.184–200.

Grover, C. 2019. Violent proletarianisation: Social murder, the reserve army of labour and social security "austerity" in Britain. *Critical Social Policy*, *39*(3), pp.335–355.

Grue, J. 2021. *I Live a Life Like Yours: A "revolutionary" memoir that rewrites our understanding of disability*. Pushkin Press.

Gulati, G., Murphy, V., Clarke, A., Delcellier, K., Meagher, D., Kennedy, H. and Dunne, C.P. 2018. Intellectual disability in Irish prisoners: Systematic review of prevalence. *International Journal of Prisoner Health*, *14*(3), pp.188–196.

Gurney, C. 2000. I ~ home: Towards a more affective understanding of home. *Proceedings of Culture and Space in Built Environments:Critical Directions/New Paradigms*, pp. 33–39

Guthrie, S., Lecko, C. and Roddam, H. 2015. Care staff perceptions of choking incidents: What details are reported? *Journal of Applied Research in Intellectual Disabilities*, *28*(2), pp.121–132.

Guttman, O.T., Lazzara, E.H., Keebler, J.R., Webster, K.L.W., Gisick, L.M. and Baker, A.L. 2021. Dissecting communication barriers in healthcare: A path to enhancing communication resiliency, reliability, and patient safety. *Journal of Patient Safety, 17*(8), pp.1465–1471.

Hall, E. 2010. Spaces of social inclusion and belonging for people with intellectual disabilities. *Journal of Intellectual Disability Research*, *54*, pp.48–57.

Hamilton, C. 2015. Sterilisation and intellectually disabled people in New Zealand: Rights, responsibility and wise counsel needed. Ko¯ tuitui: *New Zealand Journal of Social Sciences Online*, *10*(1), pp.36–45.

Hashiloni-Dolev, Y., Nov-Klaiman, T. and Raz, A. 2019. Pandora's pregnancy: NIPT, CMA, and genome sequencing – A new era for prenatal genetic testing. *Prenatal Diagnosis*, *39*(10), pp.859–865.

Hassiotis, A. 2020. The intersectionality of ethnicity/race and intellectual and developmental disabilities: Impact on health profiles, service access and mortality. *Journal of Mental Health Research in Intellectual Disabilities,13*(3), pp.171–173.

Hastings, A., Bailey, N., Bramley, G., Gannon, M. and Watkins, D. 2015. *The cost of the cuts: The impact on local government and poorer communities* (pp. 1–24). York: Joseph Rowntree Foundation.

Hatton, C. 2017. Living arrangements of adults with learning disabilities across the UK. *Tizard Learning Disability Review*, *22*(1), pp.43–50.

Hatton, C. 2024. https://chrishatton.blogspot.com/2024/11/social-care-statistics-and-adults-with.html. Retrieved 29 December 2024.

Hatzikiriakidis, K., Ayton, D., O'Connor, A., Cox, R., MacRae, A., Gulline, H. and Callaway, L. 2024. Biopsychosocial determinants of physical activity and healthy eating for people with disability living in supported accommodation: A systematic review of qualitative research. *Disability and Health Journal*, p.101618.

Haveman, M., Heller, T., Lee, L., Maaskant, M., Shooshtari, S. and Strydom, A. 2010. Major health risks in aging persons with intellectual disabilities: An overview of recent studies. *Journal of Policy and Practice in Intellectual Disabilities, 7*(1), pp.59–69.

Hellenbach, M., Karatzias, T. and Brown, M., 2017. Intellectual disabilities among prisoners: prevalence and mental and physical health comorbidities. *Journal of Applied Research in Intellectual Disabilities*, *30*(2), pp.230-24.

Hennequin, M., Faulks, D. and Roux, D. 2000. Accuracy of estimation of dental treatment need in special care patients. *Journal of Dentistry*, *28*, pp. 131–136.

Heslop, P., Blair, P., Fleming, P., Hoghton, M., Marriott, A. and Russ, L. 2013. *Confidential inquiry into premature deaths of people with learning disabilities (CIPOLD)*. Bristol: Norah Fry Research Centre.

Hill, S.E. 2015. Axes of health inequalities and intersectionality. In *Health Inequalities: Critical Perspectives*, edited by K.E. Smith and C. Bambra, 95–104. Oxford: Oxford University Press.

Hirvikoski, T., Boman, M., Tideman, M., Lichtenstein, P. and Butwicka, A. 2021. Association of intellectual disability with all-cause and cause-specific mortality in Sweden. *JAMA Network Open*, *4*(6), pp.e2113014–e2113014.

Höglund, B., Lindgren, P. and Larsson, M., 2013. Midwives' knowledge of, attitudes towards and experiences of caring for women with intellectual disability during pregnancy and childbirth: a cross-sectional study in Sweden. *Midwifery*, *29*(8), pp.950-955.

Holler, R. and Bondorevsky-Heyman, C. 2023. Social workers' perceptions of intimate relationships of people with intellectual disabilities in residential settings. *Journal of Social Work*, *23*(5), pp.821–837.

Hollins, S. 2023. *My Heart breaks; solitary confinement in hospital has no therapeutic benefit for people with a learning disability*. www.gov.uk/government/publications/independent-care-education-and-treatment-reviews-final-report-2023/baroness-hollins-final-report-my-heart-breaks-solitary-confinement-in-hospital-has-no-therapeutic-benefit-for-people-with-a-learning-disability-an Accessed on 29 December 2024.

Hough, A. 2023. Two scandals: The death of Ann Marie Smith in Australia and the Whorlton Hall scandal in Britain. *Research and Practice in Intellectual and Developmental Disabilities, 10*(1), pp.65–82.

Howden-Chapman, P. 2002. Housing and inequalities in health. *Journal of Epidemiology & Community Health*, *56*(9), pp.645–646.

Hsei, K., Rimmer, J.H. and Heller, T. 2014. Obesity and associated factors in adults with intellectual disability. *Journal of Intellectual Disability Research, 58,* pp.851–863.

Hughes, B. and Paterson, K. 1997. The social model of disability and the disappearing body: Towards a sociology of impairment. *Disability & Society, 12*(3), pp. 325–340.

Hughes-McCormack, L.A., Rydzewska, E., Cooper, S.A., Fleming, M., Mackay, D., Dunn, K., Ward, L., Sosenko, F., Barlow, F., Miller, J. and Symonds, J.D. 2022. Rates, causes and predictors of all-cause and avoidable mortality in 163 686 children and young people with and without intellectual disabilities: A record linkage national cohort study. *BMJ Open, 12*(9), p.e061636.

Humphries, K., Pepper, A., Traci, M.A., Olson, J. and Seekins, T. 2009. Nutritional intervention improves menu adequacy in group homes for adults with intellectual or developmental disabilities. *Disability and Health Journal*, *2*(3), pp.136–144.

Hussein, S.M., Soliman, W.S. and Khalifa, A.A. 2021. Benefits of pets' ownership, a review based on health perspectives. *Journal of Internal Medicine and Emergency Research, 2*, pp.1–9.

Iacono, T., Bigby, C., Unsworth, C., Douglas, J. and Fitzpatrick, P. 2014. A systematic review of hospital experiences of people with intellectual disability. *BMC Health Services Research, 14*, pp.1–8.

Ignagni E., Fudge Schormans A., Liddiard K. and Runswick-Cole K. 2016. "Some people are not allowed to love": Intimate citizenship in the lives of people labelled with intellectual disabilities. *Disability and Society*, *31*(1), pp 131–135.

Iwanaga, K., Wu, J.R., Chan, F., Rumrill, P., Wehman, P., Brooke, V.A., Avellone, L. and Taylor, J. 2021. A systematic review of systematic reviews of secondary health conditions, health promotion, and employment of people with intellectual disabilities. *The Australian Journal of Rehabilitation Counselling*, *27*(1), pp.13–40.

Jackson, R. 2011. Invited review: Challenges of residential and community care: "The times they are a-changin". *Journal of Intellectual Disability Research*, *55*(9), pp.933–944.

Jahoda, A., Banks, P., Dagnan, D., Kemp, J., Kerr, W. and Williams,V. 2009. Starting a new job: The social and emotional experi-ence of people with intellectual disabilities. *Journal of Applied Research in Intellectual Disabilities*, *22*, pp.421–425.

Jahoda, A., Kemp, J., Riddell, S. and Banks, P. 2008. Feelings about work: A review of the socio-emotional impact of supported employment on people with intellectual disabilities. *Journal of Applied Research in Intellectual Disabilities*, *21*(1), pp.1–18.

Jarrett, S. 2020. *Those they called idiots: The idea of the disabled mind from 1700 to the present day*. Reaktion Books.

Jarrett, S. 2022. The *British Journal of Learning Disabilities*: A history. *British Journal of Learning Disabilities*, *50*(2), pp.122–131.

Javaid, A., Nakata, V. and Michael, D. 2019. Diagnostic overshadowing in learning disability: Think beyond the disability. *Progress in Neurology and Psychiatry*, *23*(2), pp.8–10.

Johnson, E. 2018. *The costs of care: An ethnography of care work in two residential homes for older people*. Doctoral dissertation, Cardiff University.

Jones, C.T. 2021. " Wounds of regret": Critical reflections on competence, professional intuition, and informed consent in research with intellectually disabled people. *Disability Studies Quarterly*, *41*(2), n.p.

Julian, G. 2020. *Walking backwards into the future; involving families in investigating the deaths of learning disabled people*. Winston Churchill Memorial Trust. https://media.churchillfellowship.org/documents/Julian_G_Report_2017_Final.pdf. Accessed 29 December 2024.

Jungels, A.M. and Bender, A.A. 2015. Missing intersections: Contemporary examinations of sexuality and disability. In *Handbook of the sociology of sexualities,* edited by J. D.DeLamater and R. F. Plante (pp.169–180). Cham: Springer.

Kafer, A. 2021. After crip, crip afters. *South Atlantic Quarterly*, *120*(2), pp.415–434.

Kalman, H., Lovgren, V. and Sauer, L. 2016. Epistemic injustice and conditioned experience: The case of intellectual disability. *Wagadu: A Journal of Transnational Women's & Gender Studies*, *15*(1), p.4.

Kanner, L. 1942. Exoneration of the feebleminded. *American Journal of Psychiatry*, *99*(1), pp.17–22.

Kassee, C., Lunsky, Y., Patrikar, A. and Brown, H.K. 2023. Impact of social-, health-, and disability-related factors on pregnancy outcomes in women with intellectual and developmental disabilities: A population-based latent class analysis. *Disability and Health Journal*, *16*(2), p.101426.

Kaya, A. and Wehmeyer, M.L. 2022. A model proposal development study for adults with intellectual disabilities in Turkey compared to USA. *International Journal of Developmental Disabilities*, *70*(1), pp.89–99.

Kempton, W. and Kahn, E. 1991. Sexuality and people with intellectual disabilities: A historical perspective. *Sexuality and Disability*, *9*, pp.93–111.

Kendrick, J. 2024. Termination of parental rights on the grounds of intellectual/developmental disability: An overlooked policy and health issue. *Child & Family Social Work*, pp.1–17.

Kiani, R., Vahabzadeh, A., Hepplewhite, E.A., Abbas, M., Finnamore, T., Bhaumik, S. and Satgé, D. 2014. Overcoming challenges in diagnosing and treating cancers in people with intellectual disability: A case analysis. *Tizard Learning Disability Review, 19*(2), pp.51–58.

Kiely, E. and Warnock, R. 2023. The banality of state violence: Institutional neglect in austere local authorities. *Critical Social Policy*, *43*(2), pp.316–336.

Kinnear, D., Allan, L., Morrison, J., Finlayson, J., Sherriff, A., Macpherson, L., Henderson, A., Ward, L., Muir, M. and Cooper, S.A. 2019. Prevalence of factors associated with edentulousness (no natural teeth) in adults with intellectual disabilities. *Journal of Intellectual Disability Research, 63*(12), pp.1475–1481.

Kittay, E.F. 2001. When caring is just and justice is caring: Justice and mental retardation. *Public Culture*, *13*(3), pp.557–579.

Kittay, E.F. 2002. Not my way, Sesha, your way, Slowly.. In *Gender Struggles: Practical Approaches to Contemporary Feminism*, edited by C.L. Mui and J.S. Murphy, p.95–117. Rowman & Littlefield.

Kittay, E.F. 2009. The personal is philosophical is political: A philosopher and mother of a cognitively disabled person sends notes from the battlefield. *Metaphilosophy*, *40*(3/4), pp.606–627.

Kittay, E.F. 2020. We have seen the mutants and they are us: Gifts and burdens of a genetic diagnosis. *Hastings Center Report*, *50*, pp.S44–S53.

Kittelsaa, A. and Tøssebro, J. 2011. *Store bofellesskap for personer medutviklingshemming*. [Large group homes for people with intellectualdisabilities]. Trondheim, Norway: NTNU Social Research.

Kocman, A. and Weber, G. 2018. Job satisfaction, quality of work life and work motivation in employees with intellectual disability: A systematic review. *Journal of Applied Research in Intellectual Disabilities*, *31*, pp.1–22.

Koritsas, S. and Iacono, T. 2016. Weight, nutrition, food choice, and physical activity in adults with intellectual disability. *Journal of Intellectual Disability Research, 60*(4), pp.355–364.

Krahn, G.L. and Fox, M.H. 2014. Health disparities of adults with intellectual disabilities: What do we know? What do we do? *Journal of Applied Research in Intellectual Disabilities, 27*(5), pp.431–446.

Krahn, G.L., Hammond, L. and Turner, A. 2006. A cascade of disparities: Health and health care access for people with intellectual disabilities.*Mental Retardation and DevelopmentalDisabilities Research Review, 12*, pp.70–82.

Krasse, B. 2001. The Vipeholm Dental Caries Study: Recollections and reflections 50 years later. *Journal of Dental Research*, *80*(9), pp.1785–1788.

Krueger, C., van Heumen, L. and van den Helder, C. 2024. Self-advocacy in inclusive research. *Social Sciences*, *13*(3), p.134.

Kulick, D. 2015. When privacy and secrecy collapse into one another, bad things can happen. *Current Anthropology*, *56*(S12), pp.S241–S250.

Kumagai, A.K. and Wear, D. 2014. "Making strange": A role for the humanities in medical education. *Academic Medicine*, *89*(7), pp.973–977

Lafferty, A., McConkey, R. and Simpson, A. 2012. Reducing the barriers to relationships and sexuality education for persons with intellectual disabilities. *Journal of Intellectual Disabilities*, *16*(1), pp.29–43.

Landes, S.D., Finan, J.M. and Turk, M.A. 2022. COVID-19 mortality burden and comorbidity patterns among decedents with and without intellectual and developmental disability in the US. *Disability and Health Journal, 15*(4), p.101376.

Landes, S.D., Turk, M.A. and Lauer, E. 2020. Recommendations for accurately reporting intellectual and developmental disabilities on death certificates. *American Journal of Preventive Medicine*, *59*(6), pp.892–895.

Laugharne, R., Sawhney, I., Perera, B., Wainwright, D., Bassett, P., Caffrey, B., O'Dwyer, M., Lamb, K., Wilcock, M., Roy, A. and Oak, K. 2024. Chronic constipation in people with intellectual disabilities in the community: Cross-sectional study. *BJPsych Open*, *10*(2), p.e55.

Leary, A., Bushe, D., Oldman, C., Lawler, J. and Punshon, G. 2021. A thematic analysis of the prevention of future deaths reports in healthcare from HM coroners in England and Wales 2016–2019. *Journal of Patient Safety and Risk Management*, *26*(1), pp.14–21.

Lee, J. and Chang, J. 2021. Oral health issues of young adults with severe intellectual and developmental disabilities and caregiver burdens: A qualitative study. *BMC Oral Health, 21*, pp.1–9.

Lee, R. and Morgan, D. 1988. Sterilisation and mental handicap: Sapping the strength of the state. *Journal of Law and Society*, *15*, p.229.

Liu, Q., Adami, H.O., Reichenberg, A., Kolevzon, A., Fang, F. and Sandin, S. 2021. Cancer risk in individuals with intellectual disability in Sweden: A population-based cohort study. *PLoS Medicine, 18*(10), p.e1003840.

LoBuono, D.L., Spencer, L., Bottiglieri, J., Kientz, M., Mastrangelo, M.A., Meenar, M. and Berman, D. 2024. Evaluation of interprofessional cooking classes and home gardens in group homes. *Journal of Nutrition Education and Behavior*, *56*(10), pp.751–755.

Löfgren-Mårtenson, L. 2004. "May I?" About sexuality and love in the new generation with intellectual disabilities. *Sexuality and Disability*, *22*, pp.197–207.

Lu, S.H. and Beddoe, L. 2023. Reproductive justice and people with intellectual disabilities in Taiwan: An issue for social work. *Aotearoa New Zealand Social Work*, *35*(4), pp.144–150.

Lund, E.M. and Ayers, K.B. 2020. Raising awareness of disabled lives and health care rationing during the COVID-19 pandemic. *Psychological Trauma: Theory, Research, Practice, and Policy, 12*, pp.S210–S211.

Lunsky, Y., Durbin, A., Balogh, R., et al. 2022. COVID-19 positivity rates, hospitalizations and mortality of adults with and without intellectual and developmental disabilities in Ontario, Canada. *Disability and Health Journal, 15*, 101174.

MacPherson, H., Hall, E., Power, A. and Kaley, A. 2023. Debilitating landscapes of care and support: Envisaging alternative futures. *Social & Cultural Geography*, *24*(1), pp.140–156.

Magito-McLaughlin, D., Spinosa, T.R. and Marsalis, M.D. 2002. Overcoming the barriers: Moving toward a service model that is conductive to person-centered planning. In *Person-Centered Planning: Research, Practice and Future Directions*, edited by S.H.P.M. Vietze, pp.127–150. Baltimore, MD: Brookes Publishing.

Maguire, K., Gleeson, K. and Holmes, N. 2019. Support workers' understanding of their role supporting the sexuality of people with learning disabilities. *British Journal of Learning Disabilities,* 47, pp.59–65.

Malbon, E., Weier, M., Carey, G. and Writer, T. 2022. How personalisation programs can exacerbate socio-economic inequities: Findings from budget utilisation in the Australian National Disability Insurance Scheme. *BMC Public Health*, *22*(1), p.878.

Malli, M.A., Sams, L., Forrester-Jones, R., Murphy, G. and Henwood, M. 2018. Austerity and the lives of people with learning disabilities. A thematic synthesis of current literature. *Disability & Society*, *33*(9), pp.1412–1435.

Malouf, R., McLeish, J., Ryan, S., Gray, R. and Redshaw, M. 2017. "We both just wanted to be normal parents": A qualitative study of the experience of maternity care for women with learning disability. *BMJ Open*, *7*(3), p.e015526.

Manduchi, B., Walshe, M., Burke, É., Carroll, R., McCallion, P. and McCarron, M. 2021. Prevalence and risk factors of choking in older adults with intellectual disability: Results from a national cross-sectional study. *Journal of Intellectual & Developmental Disability*, *46*(2), pp.126–137.

Mansell, J. and Beadle-Brown, J. 2009. Dispersed or clustered housing for adults with intellectual disability: A systematic review. *Journal of Intellectual and Developmental Disability*, *34*(4), pp.313–323.

Mansell, J. and Beasley, F. 1993. Small staffed houses for people with a severe learning disability and challenging behaviour. *The British Journal of Social Work*, *23*(4), pp.329–344.

Marı'-Dell'Olmo, M., Novoa, A.M., Camprubí, L., Peralta, A., Vásquez-Vera, H., Bosch, J., Amat, J., Díaz, F., Palència, L., Mehdipanah, R. and Rodríguez-Sanz, M. 2017. Housing policies and health inequalities. *International Journal of Health Services*, *47*(2), pp.207–232.

Martin, W.J., Glass, R.I., Balbus, J.M. and Collins, F.S. 2011. A major environmental cause of death. *Science, 334*, pp.180–181.

Martino, A.S. and Perreault-Laird, J. 2019. "I don't know if I can talk about that": An exploratory study on the experiences of care workers regarding the sexuality of people with intellectual disabilities. *Disability Studies Quarterly, 39*(3), pp.1041–5718.

Martinsen, B., Harder, I. and Biering–Sorensen, F. 2008. The meaning of assisted feeding for people living with spinal cord injury: A phenomenological study. *Journal of Advanced Nursing*, *62*(5) pp.533–540.

Mason, J. and Scior, K. 2004. "Diagnostic overshadowing" amongst clinicians working with people with intellectual disabilities in the UK. *Journal of Applied Research in Intellectual Disabilities*, *17*(2), pp.85–90.

Matin, B.K., Williamson, H.J., Karyani, A.K., Rezaei, S., Soofi, M. and Soltani, S. 2021. Barriers in access to healthcare for women with disabilities: A systematic review in qualitative studies. *BMC Women's Health*, *21*, pp.1–23.

Mayes, R. and Llewellyn, G. 2012. Mothering differently: Narratives of mothers with intellectual disability whose children have been compulsorily removed. *Journal of Intellectual and Developmental Disability*, *37*(2), pp.121–130.

McCann, E., Marsh, L. and Brown, M. 2019. People with intellectual disabilities, relationship and sex education programmes: A systematic review. *Health Education Journal*, *78*(8), pp.885–900.

McCarthy, M. 1997. *The sexual experiences and sexual abuse of women with learning disabilities in institutional and community settings*. Doctoral dissertation, Middlesex University.

McCarthy, M., Bates, C., Elson, N., Hunt, S., Milne-Skillman, K. and Forrester–Jones, R. 2022. "Love makes me feel good inside and my heart is fixed": What adults with intellectual disabilities have to say about love and relationships. *Journal of Applied Research in Intellectual Disabilities*, *35*(4), pp.955–965.

McConkey, R., Keogh, F., Bunting, B., Garcia Iriarte, E. and Watson, S.F. 2016. Relocating people with intellectual disability to new accommodation and support settings: Contrasts between personalized arrangements and group home placements. *Journal of Intellectual Disabilities*, *20*(2), pp.109–120.

McConnell, A.R., Paige Lloyd, E. and Humphrey, B.T. 2019. We are family: Viewing pets as family members improves wellbeing. *Anthrozoös, 32*(4), pp.459–470.

McConnell, D. and Phelan, S. 2022. The devolution of eugenic practices: Sexual and reproductive health and oppression of people with intellectual disability. *Social Science & Medicine*, *298*, p.114877.

McGibbon, E. and Lukeman, S. 2019. Critical social justice: The moral imperative for critical perspectives in nursing. *Witness: The Canadian Journal of Critical Nursing Discourse*, *1*(1), pp.3–12.

McMahan, J. 1996. Cognitive disability, misfortune, and justice. *Philosophy and Public Affairs, 25*(1), pp.3–35.

Medina, J. 2018. Epistemic injustice and epistemologies of ignorance. In *The Routledge companion to philosophy of race*, edited by P.C. Taylor, L.M. Alcoff and L. Anderson (pp.247–260). New York: Routledge.

Medvedyuk, S., Govender, P. and Raphael, D. 2021. The reemergence of Engels' concept of social murder in response to growing social and health inequalities. *Social Science & Medicine*, *289*, p.114377.

Mee, K. and Wright, S. 2009. Geographies of belonging. *Environment and Planning A*, *41*(4), pp.772–779.

Melbøe, L. and Hardonk, S. 2022. Expanding opportunities for work and citizenship: Participation of people with intellectual disabilities in voluntary work. *Scandinavian Journal of Disability Research*, *24*(1), pp.109–121.

Meltzer, A., Robinson, S. and Fisher, K.R. 2020. Barriers to finding and maintaining open employment for people with intellectual disability in Australia. *Social Policy & Administration*, *54*(1), pp.88–101.

Merrells, J., Buchanan, A. and Waters, R. 2019. "We feel left out": Experiences of social inclusion from the perspective of young adults with intellectual disability. *Journal of Intellectual & Developmental Disability*, *44*(1), pp.13–22.

Mészáros. 2008. *Filosofia, ideologia e ciência social.* São Paulo: Boitempo.

Michael, J. 2008. *HealthCare for all: Report of the independent inquiry into access to healthcare for people with learning disabilities*. London: Independent Inquiry into Access to Healthcare for People with Learning Disabilities.

Michael, J. 2021. Potential for epistemic injustice in evidence-based healthcare policy and guidance. *Journal of Medical Ethics*, *47*(6), pp.417–422.

Michael, J. and Richardson, A. 2008. Healthcare for all: The independent inquiry into access to healthcare for people with learning disabilities. *Tizard Learning Disability Review*, *13*(4), pp.28–34.

Mikulak, M., Ryan, S., Tilley, E., Ledger, S., Davidson, L., Bebbigton, P. and Wiltshire, D. 2024. Sticky categories and their negative consequences: People with learning disabilities and 'behaviours that challenge others'. *Scandinavian Journal of Disability Research*, *26*(1), pp.110–123.

Miner, D.C., Ailey, S.H., Thompson, R.A., Squires, A., Adarlo, A. and Brown, H. 2024. "We have met the enemy and it is us": Healthcare professionals as the barrier to health equity for people with intellectual and developmental disability. *Research in Nursing & Health*, *47*(3), pp.269–273.

Mineur, T., Tideman, M. and Mallander, O. 2017. Self-advocacy in Sweden – An analysis of impact on daily life and identity of self-advocates with intellectual disability. *Cogent Social Sciences*, *3*(1), p.1304513.

Mintz, S.W. and Du Bois, C.M. 2002. The anthropology of food and eating. *Annual Review of Anthropology, 31*, pp.99–119.

Mitchell, D.T. and Snyder, S.L. 2019. Low-level agency: Disability, oppression and alternative genres of the human. In *Manifestos for the future of critical disability studies*, edited by K. Ellis, R. Garland-Thomson, M. Kent and R. Robertson (pp. 189–198). Routledge.

Mizen, L.A., Macfie, M.L., Findlay, L., Cooper, S.A. and Melville, C.A. 2012. Clinical guidelines contribute to the health inequities experienced by individuals with intellectual disabilities. *Implementation Science*, *7*, pp.1–9.

Mogensen, L.L., Drake, G., McDonald, J. and Sharp, N. 2024. Young people with intellectual disability speak out about life after school:"I want to do more in life than just… be a disability person". *Journal of Intellectual & Developmental Disability*, *49*(2), pp.121–133.

Mohamed, K. 2024. Debilitating research: Scholarship of the obvious and epistemic trauma. *African Studies*, *83*(2–3), pp. 134–151.

Monteiro, R.O., Tafla, T.L., Rodriguez, J.D.M., Teixeira, S.T., Honjo, R.S., Kim, C.A. and Teixeira, M.C.T.V. 2023. Parental attitudes and beliefs about sexuality of individuals with intellectual disability: Insights from a Brazilian sample of parents of individuals with Williams syndrome. *Journal of Applied Research in Intellectual Disabilities*, *36*(6), pp.1345–1353.

Monteleone, R. 2023. Complexity as epistemic oppression: Writing people with intellectual disabilities back into philosophical conversations. *Hypatia*, *38*(4), pp.746–759.

Morentin, R., Arias, B., Jenaro, C., Rodríguez-Mayoral, J. and McCarthy, M. 2008. Love and loving relationships in people with learning disabilities: A scientific approach. *Tizard Learning Disability Review, 13*(2), pp.33–41.

Munévar M., D.I. 2021. Dialogues between (Feminist) studies of care and (Critical) disability studies to rethink emerging activisms. In *Care and care workers: A Latin American perspective*, edited by N.A. Guimarães and H. Hirata (pp. 217–234). Switzerland: Springer.

Nevala, N., Pehkonen, I., Teittinen, A., Vesala, H.T., Pörtfors, P. and Anttila, H. 2019. The effectiveness of rehabilitation interventions on the employment and functioning of people with intellectual disabilities: A systematic review. *Journal of Occupational Rehabilitation*, *29*(4), pp.773–802.

NHS Race and Health Observatory. 2023. *We deserve better: Ethnic minorities with a learning disability and access to healthcare.* www.nhsrho.org/research/review-into-factors-that-contribute-towards-inequalities-in-health-outcomes-faced-by-those-with-a-learning-disability-from-a-minority-ethnic-community/. Accessed 29 December 2024.

NICE Quality Standard. 2015. *Annual Health Check.* www.nice.org.uk/guidance/qs101/chapter/quality-statement-2-annual-health-check. Retrieved 29 December 2024.

Nicholson, C., Finlay, W.M.L. and Stagg, S. 2023. Self-determination and co-operation in supported mealtimes involving people with severe intellectual disabilities. *Disability and Rehabilitation*, *45*(17), pp.2741–2750.

Nind, M. and Strnadová, I. 2020. Changes in the lives of people with profound intellectual and multiple disabilities. In *Belonging for People with Profound Intellectual and Multiple Disabilities*, edited by I. Strnadová and M. Nind (pp. 1–22). Routledge.

Norrie, A.W. 2018. Legal and social murder: What's the difference. *Criminal Law Review*, *7*, pp.531–542.

Northway, R., Jenkins, R. and Holland-Hart, D. 2017. Training of residential social care staff to meet the needs of older people with intellectual disabilities who develop age-related

Health problems: An exploratory study. *Journal of Applied Research in Intellectual Disabilities*, *30*(5), pp.911–921.

Nuffield Trust. 2024. www.nuffieldtrust.org.uk/sites/default/files/2024-03/Nuffield%20Trust%20-%20Learning%20disability_WEB_FINAL_1.pdf. Accessed 27 December 2024.

Nyikach, D.A. and Hansen, K.L. 2024. The lived experience of immigrant parents of disabled adolescents and young adults transitioning into adulthood: A narrative inquiry. *British Journal of Learning Disabilities, 52*(2), pp.188–198.

O'Donnell, S., Schormans, A.F. and Wilton, R. 2023. A qualitative analysis of housing and homemaking for people labelled/with intellectual disabilities in Ontario, Canada. *Housing Studies*, 40(3), pp.1–25.

O'Dowd, A. 2023. Life expectancy of minority ethnic learning disabled people is half that of white counterparts. *BMJ: British Medical Journal (Online)*, *382*, p.1713.

O'Leary, L., Cooper, S.A. and Hughes-McCormack, L. 2018. Early death and causes of death of people with intellectual disabilities: A systematic review. *Journal of Applied Research in Intellectual Disabilities*, *31*(3), pp.325–342.

ONS. 2021. www.ons.gov.uk/peoplepopulationandcommunity/birthsdeathsandmarriages/lifeexpectancies/bulletins/nationallifetablesunitedkingdom/2020to2022#:~:text=Life%20expectancy%20at%20birth%20in%20UK%20countries,-Of%20the%20four&text=Life%20expectancy%20at%20birth%20in%202020%20to%202022%20was%20estimated,and%2081.8%20years%20for%20females. Accessed 9 March 2023.

Onstot, A. 2019. Capacity to consent: Policies and practices that limit sexual consent for people with intellectual/developmental disabilities. *Sexuality and Disability*, *37*(4), pp.633–644.

Ormston, R., Eunson, J., McAteer, G. and Scotland, I.M. 2017. *Improving outcomes for people with learning disabilities: Opportunities and challenges for housing. Key findings and recommendations.* Glasgow: Scottish Commission for Learning Disability.

O'Shea, A. and Frawley, P. 2020. Gender, sexuality and relationships for young Australian women with intellectual disability. *Disability & Society*, *35*(4), pp.654–675.

O'Toole, C. 2013. Disclosing our relationships to disabilities: An invitation for disability studies scholars. *Disability Studies Quarterly*, *33*(2), n.p.

Öztürk, M.E. and Yabanci Ayhan, N.U.R.C.A.N., 2024. The relationship between the severity of intellectual and developmental disabilities (IDDs) in adults with IDDs and eating and drinking problems and nutritional status. *Journal of Intellectual Disability Research*, *68*(4), pp.325-339.

Pacheco, L., Aunos, M., Feldman, M. and McConnell, D. 2022. Reasonable efforts? Child maltreatment investigations and service referrals of parents with ascribed cognitive impairments in Canada. *Child Maltreatment*, *27*(3), pp.501–510.

Pacheco, L. and McConnell, D. 2017. Love and resistance of mothers with intellectual disability from ethnocultural communities in Canada. *Journal of Applied Research in Intellectual Disabilities*, *30*(3), pp.501–510.

Pacheco, L., More, R., Aunos, M. and Rose, R. 2024. Unfit and cast aside: Portrayals of mothering with intellectual disability in Québec court reports. *Critical Discourse Studies*, *21*(3), pp.322–340.

Pan, L. and Ye, J. 2012. Sexuality and marriage of women with intellectual disability in male-squeezed rural China. *Sexual Disability*, *30*, pp.149–160.

Paode, P. 2020. *Housing for adults with autism and/or intellectual and developmental disabilities: Shortcomings of federal programs*. The Daniel Jordan Fiddle Foundation Adult Autism Public Policy.

Patja, K., Mölsä, P. and Iivanainen, M. 2001. Cause-specific mortality of people with intellectual disability in a population-based, 35-year follow-up study. *Journal of Intellectual Disability Research*, *45*(1), pp.30–40.

Paul, E.W. 1974. The sterilization of mentally retarded persons: The issues and conflicts. *Family Planning Population Reporter, 3*(4), pp. 96–99.

Pelleboer-Gunnink, H.A., Van Oorsouw, W.M.W.J., Van Weeghel, J. and Embregts, P.J.C.M. 2017. Mainstream health professionals' stigmatising attitudes towards people with intellectual disabilities: A systematic review. *Journal of Intellectual Disability Research, 61*(5), pp.411–434.

Pérez-Curiel, P., Vicente, E., Moran, M.L. and Gomez, L.E. 2023. The right to sexuality, reproductive health, and found a family for people with intellectual disability: A systematic review. *International Journal of Environmental Research and Public Health, 20*(2), p.1587.

Perlin, M. and Lynch, A. 2016. *Sexuality, disability, and the law: Beyond the last frontier?* Springer.

Petner-Arrey, J., Howell-Moneta, A. and Lysaght, R. 2016. Facilitating employment opportunities for adults with intellectual and developmental disability through parents and social networks. *Disability and Rehabilitation*, *38*(8), pp.789–795.

Petri, G., Beadle-Brown, J. and Bradshaw, J. 2021. "Even a self-advocate needs to buy milk"–Economic barriers to self-advocacy in the autism and intellectual disability movement. *Scandinavian Journal of Disability Research*, *23*(1), pp.180–191.

Pilnick, A., Clegg, J., Murphy, E. and Almack, K. 2010. Questioning the answer: Questioning style, choice and self-determination in interactions with young people with intellectual disabilities. *Sociology of Health & Illness*, *32*(3), pp.415–436.

Pohlhaus Jr, G. 2012. Relational knowing and epistemic injustice: Toward a theory of willful hermeneutical ignorance. *Hypatia*, *27*(4), pp.715–735.

Popay, J., Whitehead, M. and Hunter, D.J. 2010. Injustice is killing people on a large scale – But what is to be done about it? *Journal of Public Health*, *32*(2), pp.148–149.

Powell, R.M., Parish, S.L. and Akobirshoev, I. 2017. The health and economic well-being of US mothers with intellectual impairments. *Journal of Applied Research in Intellectual Disabilities*, *30*(3), pp.456–468.

Power, A. and Bartlett, R. 2018. Self-building safe havens in a post-service landscape: How adults with learning disabilities are reclaiming the welcoming communities agenda. *Social & Cultural Geography*, *19*(3), pp.336–356.

Power, A., Coverdale, A., Croydon, A., Hall, E., Kaley, A., Macpherson, H. and Nind, M. 2022. Personalisation policy in the lives of people with learning disabilities: A call to focus on how people build their lives relationally. *Critical Social Policy*, *42*(2), pp.220–240.

Proctor, R.N. 1992. Genomics and eugenics: How fair is the comparison?. *Gene Mapping: Using Law and Ethics as Guides*, edited by G.J. Annas and S. Elias, pp. 57–93. Oxford: Oxford University Press.

Quilgars, D., Leishman, E., Abbott, D., Clarke, S., Cooper, B., Hodgkins, S., Scarrott, P., Pollin, A. and Beech, L. 2024. "I wouldn't change my flat for anything". Is there scope for more people with learning disabilities to rent their own homes? *British Journal of Learning Disabilities*, *52*(2), pp.362–370.

Rachman, S. 2004. Fear of contamination. *Behavior Research and Therapy*, *42*(11), pp.1227–1255.

Raphael, D., Bryant, T., Govender, P., Medvedyuk, S. and Mendly-Zambo, Z. 2022. Desperately seeking reductions in health inequalities in Canada: Polemics and anger mobilization as the way forward?. *Sociology of Health & Illness*, *44*(1), pp.130–146.

Razack, S.H. 2021. Human waste and the border: A vignette. *Law, Culture and the Humanities*, *17*(2), pp.322–334.

Redley, M. 2021. Mealtime support for adults with intellectual disabilities: Understanding an everyday activity. *Journal of Applied Research in Intellectual Disabilities*, *34*(1), pp.111–117.

Reinders, H.S. 2000. *The future of the disabled in liberal society. An ethical analysis*. Notre Dame, IN: University of Notre Dame Press.

Reiss, S., Levitan, G.W. and Szyszko, J. 1982. Emotional disturbance and mental retardation: diagnostic overshadowing. *American Journal of Mental Deficiency, 86*, pp.567–574.

Reutlinger, S. 1986. *Poverty and hunger: Issues and options for food security in developing countries. A world bank policy study*. Washington, DC: The World Bank.

Rice, J.G. and Sigurjónsdóttir, H.B. 2018. "Evidence" of neglect as a form of structural violence: Parents with intellectual disabilities and custody deprivation. *Social Inclusion*, *6*(2), pp.66–73.

Rix, J. 2023. Insults according to notions of intelligence: Perspectives from education and newsmedia. *British Journal of Learning Disabilities*, *51*(3), pp.324–333.

Roberts, C., Ditzel, N., Cooper-Moss, N., Umbleby, K. and Chauhan, U. 2024. Culturally adaptive healthcare for people with a learning disability from an ethnic minority background: A qualitative synthesis. *British Journal of Learning Disabilities*. [early online version]

Robertson, J., Beyer, S., Emerson, E., Baines, S. and Hatton, C. 2019a. The association between employment and the health of people with intellectual disabilities: A systematic review. *Journal of Applied Research in Intellectual Disabilities*, *32*(6), pp.1335–1348.

Robertson, J., Hatton, C., Emerson, E. and Baines, S. 2014. The impact of health checks for people with intellectual disabilities: An updated systematic review of evidence. *Research in Developmental Disabilities, 35*(10), pp.2450–2462.

Robertson, J., Raghavan, R., Emerson, E., Baines, S. and Hatton, C. 2019. What do we know about the health and health care of people with intellectual disabilities from minority ethnic groups in the United Kingdom? A systematic review. *Journal of Applied Research in Intellectual Disabilities*, *32*(6), pp.1310–1334.

Robinson, S. and Idle, J. 2023. Loneliness and how to counter it: People with intellectual disability share their experiences and ideas. *Journal of Intellectual & Developmental Disability*, *48*(1), pp.58–70.

Roebuck, M. 2021. Housing for people with intellectual disabilities: A scoping review. *Journal on Developmental Disabilities*, *26*(2), 1–25.

Rojas, S., Haya, I. and Lázaro-Visa, S. 2016. "My great hope in life is to have a house, a family and a daughter": Relationships and sexuality in intellectually disabled people. *British Journal of Learning Disabilities*, *44*(1), pp. 56–62.

Rose, J., Saunders, K., Hensel, E. and Kroese, B.S. 2005. Factors affecting the likelihood that people with intellectual disabilities will gain employment. *Journal of Intellectual Disabilities*, *9*(1), pp.9–23.

Rose, K.M.A. 2023. *"I want to have children, but I've got a learning disability": Understanding the reproductive and parenting imaginaries and experiences of people with learning disabilities from their perspectives and that of family members and support workers.* Doctoral dissertation, Newcastle University.

Rose, N. 1985. *The psychological complex: Psychology, politics and society 1869–1939.* London: Routledge and Kegan-Paul.

Rosich, K.J. and Hankin, J.R., 2010. Executive summary: What do we know? Key findings from 50 years of medical sociology. *Journal of Health and Social Behavior*, 51(1_suppl), pp.S1-S9.

Rossiter, K. and Clarkson, A. 2013. Opening Ontario's "saddest chapter": A social history of Huronia Regional Centre. *Canadian Journal of Disability Studies*, *2*(3), pp.1–30.

Røstad-Tollefsen, H.K., Kolset, S.O., Retterstøl, K., Hesselberg, H. and Nordstrøm, M. 2021. Factors influencing the opportunities of supporting staff to promote a healthy diet in adults with intellectual disabilities. *Journal of Applied Research in Intellectual Disabilities*, *34*(3), pp.733–741.

Røstad-Tollefsen, H.K., Kolset, S.O., Retterstøl, K., Hesselberg, H. and Nordstrøm, M. 2023. Weight reduction and dietary improvements in a cluster-randomised controlled trial for adults with intellectual disabilities. *Food & Nutrition Research*, *67*, pp. 10–29219.

Runswick-Cole, K., Smith, M., Ryan, S. and Douglas, P. 2024. Dis/entangling disability, mental health, and the cultural politics of care. *Scandinavian Journal of Disability Research*, *26*(1), pp.28–43.

Runswick-Cole, K., Ryan, S., Smith, M., Croot, L., Hatton, C., Kassa, C., Cisneros, R., Douglas, P. and The Tea and Cake Group (public involvement group who wish to stay anonymous) (under review). Tired of spinning plates: An exploration of the mental health experiences of adult/older carers of adults with learning disabilities (NIHR135080). *Health and Social Care Delivery Research.* www.journalslibrary.nihr.ac.uk/hsdr.

Ruonavaara, H. 2018. Theory of housing, from housing, about housing. *Housing, Theory and Society*, *35*(2), pp.178–192.

Rushbrooke, E., Murray, C.D. and Townsend, S. 2014. What difficulties are experienced by caregivers in relation to the sexuality of people with intellectual disabilities? A qualitative meta synthesis. *Research in Developmental Disabilities*, *35*, pp.871–886.

Russell, J., Greenhalgh, T. and Taylor, M. 2019. *Patient and public involvement in NIHR research 2006–2019: Policy intentions, progress and themes*. Oxford, UK: National Institute for Health Research.

Ryan, S. 2017. *Justice for laughing boy: Connor Sparrowhawk-A death by indifference.* London: Jessica Kingsley Publishers.

Ryan, S. 2020. *Love, learning disabilities and pockets of brilliance: How practitioners can make a difference to the lives of children, families and adults*. London: Jessica Kingsley Publishers.

Ryan, S. and O'Brien, R. 2024. Using a capability approach to explore how people with intellectual disabilities can lead flourishing lives. *Journal of Applied Research in Intellectual Disabilities*, *37*(6), p.e13299.

Ryan, S. and Runswick-Cole, K. 2009. From advocate to activist? Mapping the experiences of mothers of children on the autism spectrum. *Journal of Applied Research in Intellectual Disabilities*, *22*(1), pp.43–53.

Ryan, S., Wallace, L., Tilley, E., Tuffrey-Wijne, I., Mikulak, M., Anderson, R., Vaid, A., Bebbington, P., Keagan-Bull, R., Morrissey, E. and Martin, A. 2024a. Improving support and planning ahead for older people with learning disabilities and family carers: A mixed-methods study. *Health and Social Care Delivery Research*, *12*(16), pp.1–161.

Ryan, S., Ribenfors, F., Mikulak, M. and Coles, D. 2024b. Between epistemic injustice and therapeutic jurisprudence: Coronial processes involving families of autistic people,

people with learning disabilities and/or mental ill health. *Sociology of Health & Illness*, 1–21. https://doi.org/10.1111/1467-9566.13855.

Salmon, N., Garcia Iriarte, E., Donohoe, B., Murray, L., Singleton, G., Barrett, M. and Dillon, M. 2019. Our homes: An inclusive study about what moving house is like for people with intellectual disabilities in Ireland. *British Journal of Learning Disabilities*, *47*(1), 19–28.

Samuels, R. and Chadwick, D.D. 2006. Predictors of asphyxiation risk in adults with intellectual disabilities and dysphagia. *Journal of Intellectual Disability Research*, *50*(5), pp.362–370.

Santinele Martino, A. 2017. Cripping sexualities: An analytic review of theoretical and empirical writing on the intersection of disabilities and sexualities. *Sociology Compass*, *11*(5), e12471.

Santinele Martino, A. 2022. 'I don't want to get in trouble': A study of how adults with intellectual disabilities convert and navigate intellectual disability sexual fields. *Culture, Health & Sexuality*, *24*(9), pp.1230–1242.

Santinele Martino, A. and Schormans, A.F. 2018. When good intentions backfire: University research ethics review and the intimate lives of people labeled with intellectual disabilities. In *Forum Qualitative Sozialforschung/Forum: Qualitative Social Research 19*(3), pp.18. DEU.

Satgé, D., Axmon, A., Trétarre, B., Sandberg, M. and Ahlström, G. 2020. Cancer diagnoses among older people with intellectual disability compared with the general population: A national register study. *Journal of Intellectual Disability Research, 64*(8), pp.579–588.

Schormans, A.F., Collins, S.B., Allan, H., Allen, D.N. and Gray, N. 2024. Homeless youth with intellectual disabilities: Precarious lives and health inequalities. *British Journal of Learning Disabilities, 52*(3), pp. 477–488.

Scotch, R.K. 2009. "Nothing about us without us": Disability rights in America. *OAH Magazine of History*, *23*(3), pp.17–22.

Seeman, M.V. 2006. Starvation in psychiatric Institutions in Sweden. *International Journal of Mental Health*, *35*(4), pp.81–87.

Sen, A. 2009. Capability: Reach and limit. In *Debating global society: Reach and limits of the capability approach*, edited by E.C. Martinetti (pp.15–28). Milan: Fondazione Giangiacomo Feltrinelli.

Series, L. 2022. *Deprivation of liberty in the shadows of the institution*. Bristol University Press.

Shaw, K., Cartwright, C. and Craig, J. 2011. The housing and support needs of people with an intellectual disability into older age. *Journal of Intellectual Disability Research*, *55*(9), pp.895–903.

Sheerin, F., Fleming, S., May, P., McCallion, P., McCarron, M., Naseer, A., Lalor, G. and D'Eath, M. 2024. Challenges in care and service provision for older adults with intellectual disabilities and complex age-related conditions in Ireland. *British Journal of Learning Disabilities*, *52*(2), pp.248–259.

Sheerin, F.K., Keenan, P.M. and Lawler, D. 2013. Mothers with intellectual disabilities: Interactions with children and family services in Ireland. *British Journal of Learning Disabilities*, *41*(3), pp.189–196.

Shelton, D. 1992. Client sexual behaviour and staff attitudes: Shaping masturbation in an individual with a profound mental and secondary sensory handicap. *Journal of the British Institute of Mental Handicap* (APEX), *20*(2), pp.81–84.

Shepherd, V. 2020. An under-represented and underserved population in trials: Methodological, structural, and systemic barriers to the inclusion of adults lacking capacity to consent. *Trials*, *21*(1), pp.1–8.

Shepherd, V., Hood, K. and Wood, F. 2022. Unpacking the "black box of horrendousness": A qualitative exploration of the barriers and facilitators to conducting trials involving adults lacking capacity to consent. *Trials*, *23*(1), pp.1–25.

Shildrick, M. 2007. Contested pleasures: The sociopolitical economy of disability and sexuality. *Sexuality Research & Social Policy*, *4*, pp.53–66.

Sigurjónsdóttir, H.B. and Rice, J.G. 2017. "Framed": Terminating the parenting rights of parents with intellectual disability in Iceland. *Journal of Applied Research in Intellectual Disabilities*, *30*(3), pp.543–552.

Silverman, S.J. and Molnar, P. 2016. Everyday injustices: Barriers to access to justice for immigration detainees in Canada. *Refugee Survey Quarterly*, *35*(1), pp.109–127.

Simplican, S.C., Leader, G., Kosciulek, J. and Leahy, M. 2015. Defining social inclusion of people with intellectual and developmental disabilities: An ecological model of social networks and community participation. *Research in Developmental Disabilities*, *38*, pp.18–29.

Singer, P. 2010. "Speciesism and moral status." In *Cognitive disability and its challenge to moral philosophy*, edited by E.F. Kittay and L. Carlson (pp.331–44). Malden, MA: Wiley-Blackwell.

Siperstein, G.N., Heyman, M. and Stokes, J.E. 2014. Pathways to employment: A national survey of adults with intellectual disabilities. *Journal of Vocational Rehabilitation*, *41*(3), pp.165–178.

Sirotkin, J. 2024. *Understanding care practices and the mistreatment of disabled adults in congregate care in England*. PhD thesis, University of Leeds.

Skoss, R., Chivers, P., Arendts, G., Bulsara, C., Vithiatharan, R. and Codde, J. 2024. What supports are people with intellectual disability living in group homes provided to access health care? A case study. *British Journal of Learning Disabilities, 52*, pp.549562.

Slayter, E.M. and Jensen, J. 2019. Parents with intellectual disabilities in the child protection system. *Children and Youth Services Review*, *98*, pp.297–304.

Smith, D. 2019. Architectural sites of discrimination: Positive to negative. In *Manifestos for the future of critical disability studies*, edited by K. Ellis, R. Garland-Thomson, M. Kent and R. Robertson (pp. 142–155). Routledge.

Smith, E., Zirnsak, T.M., Power, J., Lyons, A. and Bigby, C. 2022. Social inclusion of LGBTQ and gender diverse adults with intellectual disability in disability services: A systematic review of the literature. *Journal of Applied Research in Intellectual Disabilities*, *35*(1), pp.46–59.

Smith, K.E., Hill, S. and Bambra, C. eds. 2016. *Health inequalities: Critical perspectives*. Oxford University Press.

Smith, P. 2005. Off the map: A critical geography of intellectual disabilities. *Health & Place*, *11*(2), pp.87–92.

Sobel, J. and Smith, P.S. eds. 2019. *Solitary confinement: Effects, practices, and pathways toward reform*. Oxford University Press.

Spagnuolo, N., Boulanger, J. and Ries, H. 2025. Sibling Relationships and Developmental Disability Services: From Coerced Care to Entitlement. *Disability Studies Quarterly*, *44*(2).

Spaul, S.W., Hudson, R., Harvey, C., Macdonald, H. and Perez, J. 2020. Exclusion criterion: Learning disability. *The Lancet*, *395*(10223), p.e29.

Srdanovic, B. Daw, Hayden, N., Goodley, D., Lawthom, R. and Runswick-Cole, K. 2024. Failing ethnographies as post-qualitative possibilities: reflections from critical posthumanities and critical disability studies. *Qualitative Research in Psychology*, pp.1–24.

Stancliffe, R.J., Harman, A.D., Toogood, S. and McVilly, K.R. 2011. Staffing numbers and active support: A case study. *Tizard Learning Disability Review*, *16*(3), pp.21–30.

Stefánsdóttir, G.V. and Hreinsdóttir, E.E. 2013. Sterilization, intellectual disability, and some ethical and methodological challenges: It shouldn't be a secret. *Ethics and Social Welfare*, *7*(3), pp.302–308.

Stefánsdóttir, S., Sigurjónsdóttir, H.B. and Rice, J. 2023. Weapons and tactics: A story of parents with learning disabilities maintaining family integrity. *British Journal of Learning Disabilities*, *51*(1), pp.62–69.

Stevens, A. 2004. Closer to home: A critique of British government policy towards accommodating learning disabled people in their own homes. *Critical Social Policy*, *24*(2), pp.233–254.

Strnadová, I., Johnson, K. and Walmsley, J. 2018. ".. but if you're afraid of things, how are you meant to belong?" What belonging means to people with intellectual disabilities? *Journal of Applied Research in Intellectual Disabilities*, *31*, pp.1091–1102.

Sullivan, F., Bowden, K., McKenzie, K. and Quayle, E. 2016. The close relationships of people with intellectual disabilities: A qualitative study. *Journal of Applied Research in Intellectual Disabilities*, *29*(2), 172–184.

Suuberg, A. 2020. Buck v. bell, American eugenics, and the bad man test: Putting limits on newgenics in the 21st century. *Law & Inequality*, *38*, p.115.

Svanelöv, E. and Talman, L. 2021. It is supposed to be a home: Barriers to everyday life decisions in group homes. In *Accessibility denied. Understanding inaccessibility and everyday resistance to inclusion for persons with disabilities*, edited by H. Egard, K. Hansson and D. Wasterfors (pp.159–170). Routledge.

Swope, C.B. and Hernández, D. 2019. Housing as a determinant of health equity: A conceptual model. *Social Science & Medicine*, *243*, p.112571.

Taggart, L., Mulhall, P., Kelly, R., Trip, H., Sullivan, B. and Wallén, E.F. 2022. Preventing, mitigating, and managing future pandemics for people with an intellectual and developmental disability-Learnings from COVID-19: A scoping review. *Journal of Policy and Practice in Intellectual Disabilities, 19*(1), pp.4–34.

Taghizadeh, Z., Ebadi, A., Farmahini, M. 2020. Marriage challenges of women with intellectual disability in Iran: A qualitative study. *Sexuality and Disability*, 38, pp.31–39.

Tajfel, H. 1981. *Human groups and social categories: Studies in social psychology*. Cambridge University Press.

Talbot, J. 2010. Prisoners' voices: experiences of the criminal justice system by prisoners with learning disabilities. *Tizard Learning Disability Review*, *15*(3), pp.33–41. https://doi.org/10.5042/tldr.2010.0403

Tallentire, L., Smith, M., David, L., Roberts, A., Morrow, S., Withers, P. and Smith, I. 2020. Stories of people who have attended a lesbian, gay, bisexual and trans support group in a secure intellectual disability service. *Journal of Applied Research in Intellectual Disabilities*, *33*(1), pp.17–28.

Tarasoff, L.A., Lunsky, Y., Chen, S., Guttmann, A., Havercamp, S.M., Parish, S.L., Vigod, S.N., Carty, A. and Brown, H.K., 2020. Preconception health characteristics of women with disabilities in Ontario: a population-based, cross-sectional study. *Journal of Women's Health*, *29*(12), pp.1564-1575.

Taubner, H., Tideman, M. and Staland Nyman, C. 2022. Employment sustainability for people with intellectual disability: A systematic review. *Journal of occupational rehabilitation*, *32*(3), pp.353–364.

Taylor, A. 2013. " Lives Worth Living:" Theorizing Moral Status and Expressions of Human Life. *Disability Studies Quarterly*, *33*(4).

Thomas, G.M. 2024. Can You Tell Me What Ethics Means? *The International Journal of Disability and Social Justice*, *4*(3), pp.4–22.

Thompson, V.R., Stanclife, R.J., Broom, A., Wilson, N.J. 2016. Clinicians' use of sexual knowledge assessment tools for people with intellectual disability. *Journal of Intellectual & Developmental Disability, 41*(3), pp.243–254.

Thomson, A., Bridges, S., Corrins, B., Pham, J., White, C. and Buchanan, A. 2021. The impact of physical activity and sport programs on community participation for people with intellectual disability: A systematic review. *Journal of Intellectual & Developmental Disability*, *46*(3), pp.261–271.

Thurman, W., Heitkemper, E., Hutson, T., Preston, A. and Hecht, J. 2023. "The System Tends to Scoop You Up and Spit You Out and They're Done With You": The Intersection of Intellectual/Developmental Disability and Homelessness From the Perspectives of Service Providers. *Qualitative Health Research*, *33*(11), pp.1017–1029.

Tilley, E., Strnadová, I., Danker, J., Walmsley, J. and Loblinzk, J. 2020. The impact of self-advocacy organizations on the subjective well-being of people with intellectual disabilities: A systematic review of the literature. *Journal of Applied Research in Intellectual Disabilities*, *33*(6), pp.1151-1165.

Tilly, L. 2013. 'I ain't been bothered to go': managing health problems in people with a learning disability who live without support. *Diversity and Equality in Health and Care*, *10*(4), pp.223–230.

Timmons, J.C., Hall, A.C., Bose, J., Wolfe, A. and Winsor, J. 2011. Choosing employment: Factors that impact employment decisions for individuals with intellectual disability. *Intellectual and developmental disabilities*, *49*(4), pp.285–299.

Titchkosky, T. 2003. Governing embodiment: Technologies of constituting citizens with disabilities. *Canadian Journal of Sociology/Cahiers canadiens de sociologie*, pp.517–542.

Tomsa, R., Gutu, S., Cojocaru, D., Gutiérrez-Bermejo, B., Flores, N. and Jenaro, C. 2021. Prevalence of sexual abuse in adults with intellectual disability: Systematic review and meta-analysis. *International journal of environmental research and public health*, *18*(4), p.1980.

Tøssebro, J. 2016. Scandinavian disability policy: From deinstitutionalisation to non-discrimination and beyond. *Alter*, *10*(2), pp.111–123.

Tøssebro, J., Bonfils, I.S., Teittinen, A., Tideman, M., Traustadóttir, R. and Vesala, H.T. 2012. Normalization fifty years beyond – current trends in the Nordic countries. *Journal of Policy and Practice in Intellectual Disabilities*, *9*(2), pp.134–146.

Tromans, S.J., Sawhney, I., Odiyoor, M., de Villiers, J., McCarthy, J., Boer, H., Alexander, R., Courtenay, K., Wallace, S., Gangadharan, S. and Roy, A., *et al.* 2024. Long-term segregation and seclusion for people with an intellectual disability and/or autism in hospitals: critique of the current state of affairs. *The British Journal of Psychiatry: The Journal of Mental Science*, *226*(1), pp.39–46.

Turner, G. W. and Crane, B. 2016. Pleasure is paramount: Adults with intellectual disabilities discuss sensuality and intimacy. *Sexualities*,*19*(5–6), pp.677–697.

Tyrer, F. and McGrother, C. 2009. Cause-specific mortality and death certificate reporting in adults with moderate to profound intellectual disability. *Journal of Intellectual Disability Research*, *53*(11), pp.898–904.

den Uijl, L.C., Jager, G., de Graaf, C., Waddell, J. and Kremer, S. 2014. It is not just a meal, it is an emotional experience–A segmentation of older persons based on the emotions that they associate with mealtimes. *Appetite*, *83*, pp.287–296

UK Judiciary. 2021. www.judiciary.uk/prevention-of-future-death-reports/juliet-saunders/. Accessed 1 January 2025.

UK Judiciary. 2024. www.judiciary.uk/prevention-of-future-death-reports/craig-spiby-prevention-of-future-deaths-report/. Accessed 1 January 2025.

UK Judiciary 2024a. https://www.judiciary.uk/prevention-of-future-death-reports/declan-morrison-prevention-of-future-deaths-report/

Umb Carlsson, Õ. 2021. Health-promotion intervention in a group home: Perspectives of residents, staff and rehabilitation professionals. *Journal of Intellectual Disabilities*, *25*(2), pp.210–229.

US Department of Justice and US Department of Health and Human Services. 2015b. Protecting the rights of parents and prospective parents with disabilities: technical assistance for state and local child welfare agencies and courts under Title II of the Americans with Disabilities Act and Section 504 of the Rehabilitation Act. Civil Rights Sector and Administration for Children and Families Office of Civil Rights, Washington, D.C., Available at: www.ada.gov/doj_hhs_ta/child_welfare_ta.html

Vehmas, S. 2019. Persons with profound intellectual disability and their right to sex. *Disability & Society*, *34*(4), pp.519–539.

Vehmas, S. and Mietola, R. 2021. *Narrowed Lives: Meaning, Moral Value, and Profound Intellectual Disability*. Stockholm: Stockholm University Press.

Vincent, R., Nalini, R. and Krishnakumar, K. 2024. Mothers' Perspectives on Sexual and Reproductive Health and Rights of Adolescents with Intellectual and Developmental Disabilities in Kerala, India. *Journal of Human Rights and Social Work*, *9*(1), pp.83–92.

Walmsley, J., Davies, I. and Garratt, D. 2022. 50 Years of speaking up in England – Towards an important history. *British Journal of Learning Disabilities*, *50*(2), pp.208–219.

Walmsley, J. and Jarrett, S. 2019. *Intellectual disability in the twentieth century*. Bristol: Policy Press.

Ward, N. 2011. Care ethics and carers with learning disabilities: A challenge to dependence and paternalism. *Ethics and Social Welfare*, *5*(2), pp.168–180.

White, A., Sheehan, R., Ding, J., Roberts, C., Magill, N., Keagan-Bull, R., Carter, B., Chauhan, U., Tuffrey-Wijne, I. and Strydom, A. 2023. *Learning from lives and deaths-people with a learning disability and autistic people (LEDER) report for 2022*. King's College London.

Whittle, C. and Butler, C. 2018. Sexuality in the lives of people with intellectual disabilities: A meta-ethnographic synthesis of qualitative studies. *Research in Developmental Disabilities*, 75, pp.68–81.

Whittle, E.L., Fisher, K., Srasuekbul, P. and Trollor, J., 2024. The demographic and diagnostic profile of women with intellectual disability and mental health disorder in New South Wales and patterns of service use: A data linkage study. *British Journal of Learning Disabilities*, 52(2), pp.371–384.

Wickström, M.; Larsson, M. Höglund, B. 2020. How can sexual and reproductive health and rights be enhanced for young people with intellectual disability? Focus group interviews with staff in Sweden. *Reprod. Health*, *17*, pp.1–10.

Wiesel, I. 2015. Housing for people with intellectual disabilities and the National Disability Insurance Scheme reforms. *Research and Practice in Intellectual and Developmental Disabilities*, *2*(1), pp.45–55.

Wiesel, I. and Bigby, C. 2015. Movement on shifting sands: Deinstitutionalisation and people with intellectual disability in Australia, 1974–2014. *Urban Policy and Research, 33*(2), pp.178–194.

Wiesel, I. and Bigby, C. 2016. Mainstream, inclusionary, and convivial places: Locating encounters between people with and without intellectual disabilities. *Geographical Review, 106*(2), pp.201–214.

Wiesel, I., Laragy, C., Gendera, S., Fisher, K.R., Jenkinson, S., Hill, T., Finch, K., Shaw, W. and Bridge, C. 2015. *Moving to my home: housing aspirations, transitions and outcomes of people with disability, AHURI Final Report No.246*. Melbourne: Australian Housing and Urban Research Institute.

Wigham, S., Bourne, J., McKenzie, K., Rowlands, G., Petersen, K. and Hackett, S. 2022. Improving access to primary care and annual health checks for people who have a learning disability: a multi-stakeholder qualitative study. *BMJ Open, 12*(12), p.e065945.

Willott, S., Badger, W. and Evans, V. 2020. People with an intellectual disability: under-reporting sexual violence. *The Journal of Adult Protection*, *22*(2), pp.75–86.

Wilkinson, V. J., Theodore, K. and Raczka, R. 2015. 'As normal as possible': Sexual identity development in people with intellectual disabilities transitioning to adulthood. *Sexuality and Disability*, 33(1), pp.93–105.

Willems, D.L., De Vries, J.N., Isarin, J. and Reinders, J.S. 2007. Parenting by persons with intellectual disability: an explorative study in the Netherlands. *Journal of Intellectual Disability Research*, *51*(7), pp.537–544.

Wiseman, P. and Ferrie, J. 2020. Reproductive (in)justice and inequality in the lives of women with intellectual disabilities in Scotland. *Scandinavian Journal of Disability Research*, 22(1), pp.318–329.

Wolfensberger, W., 1987. *The new genocide of handicapped and afflicted people*. Syracuse, New York: Syracuse University.

Wong, S.I. 2007. The moral personhood of individuals labeled" mentally retarded": A Rawlsian response to Nussbaum. *Social theory and practice*, *33*(4), pp.579–594.

Yee, S., Breslin, M. L., Goode, T. D., Havercamp, S. M., Horner-Johnson,W., Iezzoni, L. I. and Krahn, G. 2018. Compounded disparities: Health equity at the intersection of disability, race, and ethnicity. *The National Academies of Sciences, Engineering and Medicine*. https://dredf.org/wp-content/uploads/2018/01/Compounded-Disparities-Intersection-of-Disabilities-Race-and-Ethnicity.pdf?share=tumblrEDITORIAL|5

Yool, L., Langdon, P. E. and Garner, K. 2003. The attitudes of medium-secure unit staff toward the sexuality of adults with learning disabilities. *Sexuality and Disability*, *21*(2), pp.137–150.

Young, I. M. 2014. The five faces of oppression. In *Diversity, social justice, and inclusive excellence: Transdisciplinary and global perspectives*, edited by S.N. Asumah and M. Nagel (pp. 39–65). SUNY Press.

INDEX

FSC
www.fsc.org
MIX
Papier | Fördert
gute Waldnutzung
FSC® C083411

Kolibri 360 GmbH
Ferdinand-Jühlke-Straße 7
99095 Erfurt, Deutschland
produktsicherheit@kolibri360.de